PDQ
EPIDEMIOLOGY

Third Edition

PDQ* SERIES

Also in this series:

NORMAN, STREINER
PDQ STATISTICS

SCHLAGENHAUF-LAWLOR, FUNK-BAUMANN
PDQ TRAVELER'S MALARIA

McKIBBON, WILCZYNSKI
PDQ EVIDENCE-BASED PRINCIPLES AND PRACTICE 2/E

PDQ (Pretty Darned Quick)

PDQ
EPIDEMIOLOGY

DAVID L. STREINER, PhD
Senior Scientist, Kunin-Lunenfeld Applied Research Unit
Baycrest
Professor, Department of Psychiatry
University of Toronto
Toronto, Ontario

GEOFFREY R. NORMAN, PhD
Canada Research Chair in Cognitive
 Dimensions of Clinical Expertise
Professor of Clinical Epidemiology and Biostatistics
Assistant Dean, Programme for Educational Research
 and Development
McMaster University
Hamilton, Ontario

both of
Mc Master University Faculty of Health Sciences
Hamilton, Ontario

THIRD EDITION

with 43 illustrations

2009
People's Medical Publishing House—USA
Shelton • Connecticut

People's Medical Publishing House—USA
2 Enterprise Drive, Suite 509
Shelton, CT 06484
Tel: 203-402-0646
Fax: 203-402-0854
E-mail: info@pmph-usa.com

PMPH-USA

09 10 11 12/PMPH/6 5 6 5 4 3 2 1

ISBN 978-1-60795-022-6
Printed in China by People's Medical Publishing House

Sales and Distribution

Canada
McGraw-Hill Ryerson Education
Customer Care
300 Water St
Whitby, Ontario L1N 9B6
Canada
Tel: 1-800-565-5758
Fax: 1-800-463-5885
www.mcgrawhill.ca

Foreign Rights
John Scott & Company
International Publisher's Agency
P.O. Box 878
Kimberton, PA 19442
USA
Tel: 610-827-1640
Fax: 610-827-1671

Japan
United Publishers Services Limited
1-32-5 Higashi-Shinagawa
Shinagawa-ku, Tokyo 140-0002
Japan
Tel: 03-5479-7251
Fax: 03-5479-7307
Email: kakimoto@ups.co.jp

United Kingdom, Europe, Middle East, Africa
McGraw Hill Education
Shoppenhangers Road
Maidenhead
Berkshire, SL6 2QL
England
Tel: 44-0-1628-502500
Fax: 44-0-1628-635895
www.mcgraw-hill.co.uk

Singapore, Thailand, Philippines, Indonesia,
Vietnam, Pacific Rim, Korea
McGraw-Hill Education
60 Tuas Basin Link
Singapore 638775

Tel: 65-6863-1580
Fax: 65-6862-3354
www.mcgraw-hill.com.sg

Australia, New Zealand
Elsevier Australia
Tower 1, 475 Victoria Avenue
Chatswood NSW 2067
Australia
Tel: 0-9422-8553
Fax: 0-9422-8562
www.elsevier.com.au

Brazil
Tecmedd Importadora e Distribuidora
de Livros Ltda.
Avenida Maurilio Biagi 2850
City Ribeirao, Rebeirao, Preto SP
Brazil
CEP: 14021-000
Tel: 0800-992236
Fax: 16-3993-9000
Email: tecmedd@tecmedd.com.br

India, Bangladesh, Pakistan, Sri Lanka, Malaysia
CBS Publishers
4819/X1 Prahlad Street 24
Ansari Road, Darya, New Delhi-110002
India
Tel: 91-11-23266861/67
Fax: 91-11-23266818
Email:cbspubs@vsnl.com

People's Republic of China
PMPH
Bldg 3, 3rd District
Fangqunyuan, Fangzhuang
Beijing 100078
P.R. China
Tel: 8610-67653342
Fax: 8610-67691034
www.pmph.com

*To two individuals who have provided
comfort and solace in the difficult times
and added to our pleasure in the good times—
Jim Beam and Johnny Walker.*

Contents

Preface

Welcome to the wonderful world of epidemiology. Just when you figured that you had mastered the mysteries of pulmonary blood flow, cardiac rhythms, electrolyte balance, gut motility, and cerebral anatomy, along came this strange guy in a tweed jacket muttering formulas, statistics, and foreign-sounding words like "relative risk," "positive predictive value," and "Mantel-Haenzel chi-square." He didn't look like a scientist: no dirty lab coat, scientific calculator, or long hair. He didn't look like a real doctor either: no clean lab coat, stethoscope, or designer length hair. Yet he had the arrogance to claim that he is both a clinician *and* a scientist—he is a clinical epidemiologist. Amid the hushed silence in the room you can overhear desperate whispers of, "What in the world is a clinical whatever-it-is-ologist?"

More particularly, why, in a world already overpopulated by physiologists, pharmacologists, pathologists, gerontologists, nephrologists, cardiologists, neurologists, and a dozen other relatively legitimate art forms, do we need yet another -ologist?

The answer, it seems, is that somewhere in that complex, compartmentalized world that lays claim to the human body as an object of study, common sense got lost in the shuffle. The reality is that, despite a tremendous explosion in biomedical science, we still know embarrassingly little about the workings of ourselves. No one knows the cause of most diseases or the cure for that matter. No one can lay claim to the crystal ball that will predict accurately who, among a group of cancer or postmyocardial infarction patients, will survive a year. As a result, there is a considerable gap between the exact findings of the laboratory and the uncertain world of clinical medicine. This leaves enormous room for the dissemination of well-intended but useless tests, therapies, or theories.

Some examples may illustrate the point:

1. As we have been told by the media on countless occasions, dioxin is about the most lethal chemical known. A tiny dose causes mice to curl up and die; dioxins are teratogenic, mutagenic, and carcinogenic in the lab. Yet despite all the tons of Agent Orange dumped over Vietnam and

some large spills in places like Seveso, Italy, there is no evidence that they are a significant human carcinogen.

2. Conversely, cigarette smoking is easily the most lethal human carcinogen, measured in the number of lives lost. Yet it was long after good scientific evidence from human studies convinced everyone (except tobacco farmers and cigarette manufacturers) that it caused cancer that scientists were able to induce cancers in mice in the laboratory.

3. Clofibrate was a very popular lipid-reducing agent in the mid-1960s. There was abundant laboratory evidence that it would work as claimed. Unfortunately, later randomized trials proved that the drug killed more people than it saved.

4. We like to think that the days of patent medicines and snake oil salesmen have passed. (However, one visit to your local drugstore to peruse the over-the-counter antiarthritis drugs, none of which contains anything more than aspirin and all of which cost 10 times as much, should dispel that myth.) Nevertheless, mainstream medicine is still susceptible to the legitimate and honest claims of success of new therapies based on experience with few patients. Many of these therapies are eventually proved to have no value. One case in point is gastric freezing. There were a number of case reports, involving a total of about 1,500 patients, that indicated that it would cure ulcers. It was only later that trials demonstrated that the procedure was useless.

5. Whatever happened to tonsillectomies? It seems as if five out of six adults over the age of 40 had their tonsils removed in childhood, but very few of our children have to endure this agony. Credit for the turnaround belongs to one of the neater epidemiologic studies. It was common wisdom in those days that roughly half of all kids needed their tonsils removed. These investigators started with about 400 kids who still had their tonsils and shipped them around to a group of respected physicians. Sure enough, 45 percent of tonsils had to go. The researchers removed these "diseased" kids from the study and sent the remaining ones around again (to different physicians, of course). This time 46 percent of the tonsils were slated to go. Now, the kids who were left (who had been judged healthy by two sets of physicians by this time) were marched before a third group of doctors. Want to guess how many were said to need tonsillectomies? You got it—44 percent.

These examples nicely illustrate the role of epidemiology these days—it comfortably fills the gaping chasm between the scientific wisdom of the wet laboratory and the clinical wisdom of the ward. The good news is that it isn't all that hard. Despite the fancy terminology, epidemiology is, above all, the science of common sense. (Its bedmate, biostatistics, isn't quite so straightforward. To decipher the arcane logic of statisticians, we heartily recommend another book in the *PDQ* series—*PDQ Statistics*. We're biased, of course, because we wrote it.)

The intent of this book is to translate the terminology of epidemiology into street talk, so that, we hope, the common sense of the methods will emerge. It's laid out a bit like a dictionary. Topics are grouped in logical rather than alphabetic order, so it would behoove you to tackle one section at a time. Chapter 1 is an introduction that goes into more detail about what epidemiology can and cannot do. Chapter 2 goes into depth about classical epidemiology, and Chapter 3 talks about experimental designs. Chapter 4 examines the issues in measurement, Chapter 5 provides the criteria of causation, and Chapter 6 explores some of the ethical problems that researchers must address.

At the end of the third, fourth, and fifth chapters, we've provided guides to help you determine whether articles that you have come across have made some basic mistakes in design or reasoning. As in our previous book, *PDQ Statistics,* we've called these illustrations "Convoluted Reasoning or Antiintellectual Pomposity Detectors," which we've abbreviated as "C.R.A.P. Detectors." This was done solely for the laudable purpose of conserving space, and anyone who reads any other meaning into this name reveals a low sense of humor; such people should enjoy this book.

We can't guarantee that your graduate degree will be mailed after you finish this book. Nevertheless, we hope that you will find all the fancy words a bit less intimidating.

PREFACE TO THE THIRD EDITION

Compared to such ancient fields as surgery and dentistry, epidemiology is the new kid on the block. Although we somewhat tongue-in-cheek trace its roots back to the Bible (that other one, not the one you're holding right now), it didn't really get its start until the middle of the 19th century. So it can probably be said that the field is in its middle years now, and as many people find to their dismay, middle age brings spread. In the case of epidemiology, that spread has been caused by incorporating concepts and techniques from other areas, such as meta-analysis and quasi-experimental designs. Meta-analysis got its start in the mid-1970s in psychology, and since then has become a growth industry in the health sciences. We counted 20 articles using the keyword "meta-analysis" that were published in 1980, and nearly 4,000 in 2007—a rate of increase that would be the envy of any investment fund manager (although as we're writing this, just breaking even would make them incredibly happy). Similarly, clinical epidemiology was at first almost synonymous with "randomized controlled trial." As the field has matured, though, many have come to realize that many interventions, and many other kinds of research questions, cannot be evaluated in this way, and that even the stalwarts of classical epidemiology—case-control and cohort studies—have their limitations. Again, concepts from other fields (evaluation, psychology, and education) have filled the gap, in this case with quasi-experimental designs.

So to keep up with the changes, we have added sections that explain both of these sets of techniques. At the same time, we have expanded the section on the RCT, adding more variants to the mix, such as patient-preference designs, and going into more detail about concepts such as the differences between efficacy and effectiveness trials and whom to count. The section on measurement has been brought into line with the more recent conceptualizations of reliability and validity; there aren't different "types" of validity, such as criterion or content validity, but rather that everything is subsumed under *construct validity*. We have also added a section on screening, discussing when it may actually do more harm than good. Finally, we realized that some of our examples carried over from the first edition had become somewhat (or terribly) dated, so those have been brought up to date, and new data introduced for the examples that stayed.

What hasn't changed, we hope, is the style. "Humor" shouldn't refer only to black bile, yellow bile, blood, and phlegm; we feel it should be an integral component of all books, and the drier the subject, the more important it is. Nothing is drier than epidemiology (except for statistics or a good martini), so it is vitally important here, and we hope we deliver it in generous doses.

David L. Streiner
Geoffrey R. Norman

REFERENCES

Bakwin H: Pseudodoxia pediatrica, *N Engl J Med* 232:691–697, 1945.

Miao LL: Gastric freezing: an example of the evaluation of medical therapy by randomized clinical trials. In Bunker JP, Barnes BA, Mosteller F, editors: *Costs, risks, and benefits of surgery,* New York, 1977, Oxford University Press.

Oliver MF, Heady JA, Morris JN: WHO cooperative trial on primary prevention of ischaemic heart disease using clofibrate to lower serum cholesterol: mortality follow-up, *Lancet* 2:379–385, 1980.

Serum dioxin in Vietnam-era veterans—preliminary report, *Morb Mortal Wkly Rep* 36:470–475, 1987.

PDQ
EPIDEMIOLOGY

1

Introduction to Epidemiology

WHAT IT IS

Contrary to popular belief, epidemiology is *not* the study of skin diseases—the root word is *epidemic*, not *epidermis*. And if you really want to impress your friends, tell them that the word *epidemic* itself comes from the Greek *epi*, meaning "among," and *demos*, meaning "the people." One scholar defined epidemiology as "the study of the distribution and determinants of health-related states and events in populations and the application of this study to the control of health problems," which no doubt is about as clear and self-evident as a mortgage contract.

For many years, if epidemiology was taught at all in medical schools (oops, that should be "health sciences centers" or some such euphemism), it was put in the same category as gross anatomy or biochemistry—one of those subjects you had to study so the old crock teaching it could keep a job but probably of no use in the real world. Fortunately, recent history is on our side. Before Legionnaires' disease came along in 1976, the only people who had ever heard of epidemiology were other epidemiologists. Now that we have toxic shock syndrome (TSS), acquired immunodeficiency syndrome (AIDS), Agent Orange, repetitive strain injuries, the Gulf War syndrome, reactions to silicone breast implants, sick building syndrome, and leukemias purportedly caused by high-tension wires, epidemiology is second on the list of careers advocated by every high school guidance counselor (coming after high school guidance counselor).

We still haven't told you what epidemiology really is, so we should get down to it. Alderson states that epidemiology includes four different types of studies: descriptive, hypothesis testing, interventional, and methodologic. **Descriptive studies** address questions like, "Who is most likely to develop AIDS?" or "What do the outbreaks of Legionnaires' disease have in common?" or "Is there any association between kids who live near high-tension wires and the development of anemia?" This type of research (1) looks at the world as it is without trying to change it, (2) relies on existing data, such as the census, or (3) uses surveys of large groups of people to collect the information.

Once we have (or at least think we have) a good description of what's related to what, we can ask more specific questions and move into the **hypothesis testing** phase. For example, if we suspect that the chances of developing breast cancer may be related to the intake of fatty foods, we can see whether countries that have low-fat diets also have a low prevalence of cancer and whether this prevalence is related to fat intake. Similarly, if we think that Legionnaires' disease is caused by stagnant water in cooling systems, we can immediately test for water purity as soon as we hear about an outbreak. Again, we are pretty much leaving the world alone and "simply" gathering more focused information—information that can support or refute a specific hypothesis.

If after this stage our hypotheses are still viable (it's amazing how few can survive the bright light of data), we may want to move on to the third stage, which is **intervention studies**. Now finally we're getting a chance to change things. Rather than simply observing the relationship between low-density lipoprotein (LDL) cholesterol and coronary heart disease, we can do a study to see whether lowering cholesterol in one group of people leads to a lower death rate than in people belonging to the group we leave alone. Notice that we're still using hypothesis testing as with the second stage but with an added wrinkle—we now have more control over some of the variables.

Each of these types of epidemiologic research may require us to develop methods to gather the necessary data or carry out the intervention. For example, we were once interested in seeing whether social support could ameliorate the adverse effects of stress on physical illness. To do so, though, we first had to develop an appropriate measure of social support because none of the existing ones met our needs. We also had to do a pilot study to determine the best way of ensuring compliance among the subjects completing health diaries (and returning them to us) during a 2-year span. These **methods studies** not only helped us carry out the major study but they also led to a number of publications, which didn't do our careers any harm (we think).

Thus epidemiology covers a broad spectrum, overlapping with demography at one end, encompassing survey research in the middle, and looking much like experimental medicine at the other end. The common thread uniting all of these activities is a *focus on groups of people* rather than on individuals, molecules, cells, or mice.

Until relatively recently the field of epidemiology was more limited, covering only the first two aspects, descriptive studies and hypothesis testing. For this reason, studies of these types are sometimes called **classical epidemiology** or **big-E epidemiology**. Now the field includes **clinical epidemiology**, which got its start with the first modern clinical trial in the 1950s, although as we'll see, the ancestry of studies of health effects of different regimens on humans can actually date back 3500 years or so. Modern epidemiology incorporates both classical and clinical epidemiology. As Cassel noted, epidemiology is an example of a discipline that has expanded beyond its initial boundaries (sort of like the Sahara Desert and our waistlines).

TRENDS IN EPIDEMIOLOGY

We like to think of the development of science as following a straight path. First, some of our primitive ancestors made an astute observation, such as how summer rain storms are often accompanied by thunder and lightning. This led to the hypothesis that a god on Mount Olympus was throwing things at us, which was later replaced by a correct theory (correct because it's what we believe today). Based on our improved knowledge, we are now able to intervene, such as by seeding clouds to produce rain when we want it or to prevent tornadoes when we don't want them. Thus we move from observing and hypothesizing (classical epidemiology) to intervening and improving (clinical epidemiology).

Comforting as this picture is, it doesn't correspond too closely with reality. As we'll see in the next chapter, epidemiology did in fact start with observation and hypothesis generation. This occurred during what has been called the *Age of Pestilence and Famine*, when the major health threats were infectious diseases, such as tuberculosis (TB), cholera, influenza, the plague, and so forth. This time was characterized by high and variable mortality rates, very low life expectancy, and a slow growth (if any) in the population. Starting in the 18th century, at least in developed countries, we entered into the first **epidemiologic transition**, usually called the *Age of Receding Pandemics* (a term we'll define in the next chapter). During this stage, many infectious diseases were either completely wiped out (e.g., smallpox) or contained (e.g., polio, TB). Epidemics became less frequent, resulting in greater life expectancy, increased population growth, and less variation in the mortality rate. In a very influential book, McKeown said that at least initially, this was due primarily to an improvement in living standards, which accompanied an increase in income, and had little to do with medicine. For example, deaths in England and Wales from respiratory diseases started declining many years before we had an effective treatment for TB; indeed, before we even knew what caused it. This transition occurred later in developing countries, such as China and Mexico, and was due primarily to effective disease control, rather than individual income. But, no good deed ever goes unpunished. As life expectancy increased, we entered into the next epidemiologic transition, the *Age of Degenerative and Man-Made Diseases* (although in this era of political correctitude, it should probably be renamed as *Degenerative and Person-Made Diseases*). We are now dealing with problems that were rarely seen previously, because people didn't live long enough to develop them (e.g., dementia and glaucoma) or are caused by "lifestyle" behaviors, such as smoking cigarettes and munching on potato chips while watching the 958th football game of the season. We could also call this the *Age of Useful Interventions*, because we can now evaluate which medicines, surgical treatments, and behavioral interventions actually produce more success stories than failures.

So far, so good; epidemiology is following the pattern that we would like to see. But at the same time that we're moving into this latest age, we are suddenly rediscovering outbreaks of infectious diseases in the developed world. Within the past few years, a new Hantavirus outbreak occurred in the mid-western United States, and it took all the tools of the classical epidemiologists to trace it to the droppings of cute-looking mice. Similarly, TB, which we thought was almost completely wiped out through a combination of better drugs and improved housing, has come back in a more treatment-resistant form to attack people living in the city cores and especially people with compromised immunologic systems as a result of human immunodeficiency virus (HIV) infection. Even more recently, we've seen outbreaks of new infectious diseases, such as Severe Acute Respiratory Syndrome (SARS) and the avian flu; and in Walkerton, Ontario, in May 2000, seven people died and about 2,500 people came down with severe diarrhea and gastrointestinal symptoms from a well contaminated with a dangerous strain of *E. coli* bacteria. So it's back to making observations about acute infections and testing hypotheses.

In many ways, this is similar to the prediction made in about 1900 by an eminent professor who decreed that, given the natural history of physics, approximately 3 more years of research would suffice to solve all the remaining problems. His major mistake was underestimating the survival instinct of researchers. Epidemiologists have been equally adaptive, moving from infections to chronic diseases to drug trials (where the real money is). They have been just as adaptable by moving back to studying infectious and chronic diseases as these have reemerged as major problems (thus guaranteeing many more years of employment).

CURRENT APPLICATIONS OF EPIDEMIOLOGY

In case you're still confused about what this marvelous new (old) science is all about, this section provides some topical examples of epidemiologic studies and a hint of some of the techniques that were used.

Identifying the Cause of a New Syndrome

The late 1970s saw a number of cases of menstruating women who experienced a cluster of symptoms including fever, hypotension, and a rash, followed by desquamation (a fancy term that simply means "peeling") on the hands, soles, fingers, or toes. Within a short time, 50 cases had been reported to the Centers for Disease Control and Prevention (CDC) in Atlanta, and three women had died. Two questions required an urgent response: (1) Is this a new syndrome? and (2) What is causing it?

Through an examination of the records, it was determined that these 50 cases were presenting a new clinical entity, described by Langmuir as a "distinct clinical syndrome of marked severity and considerable clinical specificity." This was labeled TSS. Let's take a closer look at the history of this disorder because it nicely highlights many of the steps used to discover the cause of a problem and, in this case at least, the interventions needed to alleviate it.

The first step was **passive surveillance**. Neither the CDC nor the local public health agencies initially went out looking for cases of this new disorder. Rather, they relied on reports submitted voluntarily by local physicians and other agencies. The major advantage of passive surveillance is that no single agency is always on the lookout for an outbreak of something, especially if they don't know what that something is or if indeed anything is breaking out at all. There is the hope that any new and especially any potentially dangerous syndrome will be noticed by the front-line people (e.g., family physicians, laboratory workers, community health nurses) and reported to the health office. The downside of remaining passive is that reporting is extremely sporadic; a person first has to notice that something is amiss and then take the time and effort to report this to some agency. So passive surveillance can alert people that *something* is happening, but it can't really say how big the problem is or where the hot-spots are. This is exactly what happened with TSS; the CDC learned that there was an outbreak of a possibly new disorder, but it was still in the dark regarding the outbreak's magnitude or what may be causing it.

Perhaps the most widely used versions of passive surveillance are published **case reports** and **case series**. Grimes and Schulz describe the case report as "the least publishable unit in the medical literature"; a report of a single patient with what—at least to the author—appears to be a new syndrome. Although frequently derided as non-scientific and something published "simply to enliven the generally drab medical literature," there have been a number of disorders that were first described in case reports— the "elephant man" written up by Frederick Treves; Paul Broca's description of aphasia due to lesions in the ventroposterior region of the frontal lobes; and William MacIntyre's discovery of multiple myeloma. When a number of individual cases have been aggregated into a single article, it's called a **case series**. This can be the first signs of an adverse drug reaction or even an epidemic, as happened with asthma patients being killed by their nebulizers containing isoproterenol in the 1960s; AIDS in Los Angeles in 1981; and *eosinophilia myalgia* due to contaminated L-tryptophan (bought at "natural" food stores) in 1989. On the other hand, they can simply reflect the co-occurrences of relatively rare events which happened by chance, but are then attributed to some underlying "cause." This happened with autism and childhood vaccinations, and with silicone breast implants and systemic lupus. Given the large number of people who have been vaccinated or have had their breasts enhanced (not usually at the same time, though), it's inevitable that some will develop a given disorder. Putting them all in one case series makes it look like cause-effect relationship. But, without a comparison group, it's impossible to determine whether the prevalence of the disorder is the same in the group that didn't have the intervention (it is, in both cases). In the meantime, a lot of mischief can be done—kids not receiving their inoculation because of the parents' fears of autism in the one case, and the bankruptcy of a company in the other.

Once an agency suspects that a problem may exist, it usually then relies on **active surveillance**. The agency becomes more active and tries to solicit complete reporting of the new syndrome by contacting family physicians, medical officers of health, or laboratories. Depending on the degree of cooperation received, it's now possible to get a better handle on the magnitude of the problem and perhaps to develop some hypotheses about what may be causing the outbreak. The CDC and state agencies begin to look for cases, such as TSS, using active surveillance by both getting front-line workers to report to them and examining the charts and discharge codes in selected hospitals.

To sharpen their hypotheses, the agencies began a series of studies in which people who had TSS were compared with those who didn't (these are called **case control studies**, and we'll discuss them in more depth in Chapter 3). They were particularly interested in tampon use because the previous observations led them to believe that TSS may be associated with menses. These case control studies, especially those conducted by the CDC, finally nailed down the cause. In their first study, all 52 cases used tampons, but only 85% of the control women did. In the second study, women who used the Rely brand of tampons were almost eight times more likely to develop TSS than women who used other brands. Finally, it was found that other brands were involved and that the culprit was the increased absorbency of the "new and improved" versions (so much for the advantages of new and improved anything).

Now to the intervention. In Figure 1-1, we see a sharp increase in TSS cases until 1980. At that point, Rely was voluntarily withdrawn from the marketplace, resulting in a dramatic decrease in reported cases. For the next 4 years, the proportion of women using very high-absorbency products dropped from 42% to 18% and down to 1% by 1986, and the most absorbent tampons, those made with polyacrylate, were taken off the market in 1985. The effect of these changes on the number of reported cases is striking.

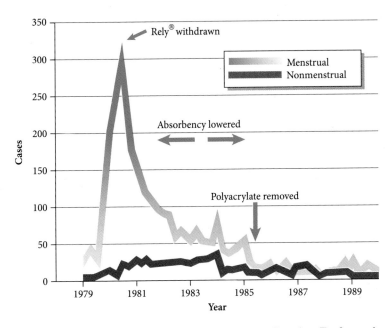

Figure 1-1. Incidence of toxic shock syndrome cases per year. (Data from The Centers for Disease Control and Prevention.)

TSS hasn't completely disappeared, because it is caused by the staphylococcus organism, not by tampons. There are still a few cases every year, usually as a result of surgery, so it occurs in men as well as in non-menstruating women. On the whole, though, this example demonstrates the strength of epidemiologic methods. Even given a relatively rare condition, such as TSS, associated with a common practice, such as tampon use, it could nonetheless be established that high-absorbency tampons were the culprit and that removing them from store shelves could stop the outbreak.

Assessing the Risks Associated with a Harmful Exposure

Epidemiologic methods can be used to assess the risks to health that result from exposure to noxious agents. For example, with the worldwide use of nuclear reactors to generate power, the public, the nuclear power industry, and nuclear regulatory bodies are all interested (obviously for different reasons) in determining the risks associated with exposure to the radioactive emissions resulting from a nuclear "accident" (a benign term for a malignant condition). These interests are not merely hypothetical or academic. In 1957 the first documented nuclear "accident," or substantial release of radioactivity from a nuclear power plant, occurred when a reactor caught fire at Sellafield on the Irish coast of Great Britain; in 1979 a nuclear accident occurred when a reactor was damaged at Three Mile Island; and in 1986 the most severe nuclear accident to date occurred at Chernobyl, in the former Union of Soviet Socialist Republics (USSR), when the graphite core of a reactor caught fire and caused the rupture or "meltdown" of fuel rods and the release of radioactive fission products into the atmosphere. Winds distributed the radioactive particles over large areas of Europe and the Northern Hemisphere.

It is of obvious importance to determine the immediate and long-term risks to the populations in the immediate vicinity of the nuclear accident and to those farther from the reactor (in other regions or countries). Fortunately, there is already a great deal of evidence available about the risks of cancer, childhood leukemia, birth defects, and so forth that result from exposure to high-level and low-level radiation. By far the most extensive source of human evidence resulted from careful follow-up during the past 5 decades of the survivors of the Hiroshima and Nagasaki bombings. The basic strategy is to document, as carefully as possible, the radiation exposure of each individual and then to compare the rate of onset of various diseases at different levels, from no exposure to a high level. Other sources of evidence derive from the documented exposure of soldiers in the atom bomb tests of the 1950s, workers at the shipyards where nuclear submarines were serviced, populations exposed to the fall-out clouds in Utah and Nevada, atomic workers, and even kids (now in their '60s) who put their feet in fluoroscopy machines at the local shoe store.

Based on this evidence the scientists have predicted that there might be as many as 39,000 additional cancer deaths worldwide during the next 50 years. Because there are expected to be approximately 630 million deaths from cancer during the same period, the increase will not be detectable. Within the former USSR, estimates range from 5,000 to 50,000 excess deaths against a background of 9.5 million cancer deaths; again, the difference will not be statistically significant. However, among the 24,000 people who lived within 15 km of the reactor site, the estimated excess number of cancers is 13, which raises the total to 624; this will be statistically detectable. Interestingly, actual data collected since that time tell a different story. One huge study of childhood leukemia involved national registries of all the European countries. There were 3,679 observed cases versus 3,533 expected cases—a relative risk of 1.04. There was no association between risk and exposure, leading the authors to discount any causal connection between the observed increase in leukemia and Chernobyl radiation. Another study looked at thyroid nodules (an early indicator of cancer from radiation exposure), comparing people in highly exposed villages near the reactor and control villages. Again, no significant increase. Well, Chernobyl celebrated its 20th anniversary in 2006, accompanied by the release of a WHO report. According to estimates, there was a substantial excess of childhood thyroid cancer, although this has a 98.8% cure rate, so resulted in eight deaths. There were 134 emergency workers involved in the immediate cleanups; 28 died of acute radiation sickness in 1986, and 19 more between 1987 and 2004. Of the 200,000 "liquidators" involved in the later cleanup, it is estimated there will eventually be 22% overall cancer mortality vs. a normal 21%, although this has not been observed. According to the report, "Total mortality among Russian emergency workers does not differ in a statistically significant way from ... the whole Russian population" (p. 106). In the population within 30 km. (20 mi.) of Chernobyl and those in the "seriously contaminated zone," encompassing 400,000 people, the study has not "revealed any strong evidence for radiation-induced increase in general population mortality . . . caused by leukemia, solid cancers (other than thyroid), and non-cancer diseases" (p. 107). The best projected estimate is an increase of about 1,750 cancers, against a background of 65,000. Of course, these figures remain estimates into the future; observed deaths attributable to radiation are much lower. In any case, they are substantially lower than the estimates of 50,000 or more in the early writings. One thing has significantly increased since the accident—the number of articles about Chernobyl. A Medline search retrieved more than 3,400 articles since 1986.

Epidemiologic studies have played a fundamental role in demonstrating the risk to health from such domestic exposures as smoking, nitrates in food, high dietary cholesterol, and occupational exposure to factors like asbestos, lead, and rubber. Conversely, epidemiologic methods have shown that there exists little evidence of harm from other exposures. For example, formaldehyde release from urea formaldehyde foam insulation, "yellow rain" in Southeast Asia, video display terminals, and silicone breast implants have all, at one time or another, been featured prominently in news reports. Subsequent epidemiologic investigations, however, have revealed little in the way of measurable health problems from these highly publicized cases.

In turn the identification of these risk factors may lead to the identification and effective treatment of those already exposed (e.g., screening and treatment for hypertension) and can suggest strategies for prevention (e.g., guarantees of adequate income for single-parent families to prevent some childhood psychiatric disorders).

How to Determine Whether a Treatment Is Effective

You are a 33-year-old mother of two children. Last week you noticed a small lump in one breast. With considerable apprehension, you made an appointment with your family physician. Today the doctor announced that your fear was justified; the lump is malignant. Your physician recommends total mastectomy (a surgical procedure that involves amputation of the breast but not of the underlying muscle and lymph nodes) and assures you that if you have this procedure, your condition is almost certainly curable. A friend of yours had a diagnosis of breast cancer more than 1 year ago, and her physician removed just enough tissue to eliminate the tumor (lumpectomy) and gave her radiation therapy. You are frightened by the disease and want the treatment that will be most effective in preventing a recurrence of the cancer. On the other hand, you are devastated at the prospect of losing your breast. Clearly, if the treatment your friend had is as effective as total mastectomy, it would be your treatment of choice.

How do you decide what to do? Being human, you would likely seek out other friends who have gone through the procedures. In the absence of friends, there are still the journals *Ladies' Home Journal* and *Consumer Reports* (the latter actually does a good job of reporting medical research). However, if you or your close friends had access to MEDLINE and a medical library, there is the option of seeking out the original articles.

Clinical epidemiology figures prominently in the review. The methods of clinical epidemiology have contributed much to the assessment of the effectiveness of particular treatments. In the case of breast cancer the primary issue is whether there is any greater chance of survival with total mastectomy versus lumpectomy. The question of effectiveness must be clearly defined, including both the specifics of the treatment and the particular cases to which it is applied. For example, lumpectomy may be just as effective in treating early stage breast cancer, whereas it may well be ineffective in treating later stage breast cancer after the malignant cells have spread beyond the immediate area.

Some additional concerns may relate to the side effects. If there is no difference in survival between two treatments, it becomes a tradeoff between the short-term discomfort from chemotherapy or hair loss from radiation and the disfigurement and disability from the loss of the breast. An approach that may help when examining side effects is to seek out information about the differences in psychologic adjustment after total mastectomy versus lumpectomy and radiation therapy.

The best data on whether a treatment does more good than harm come from an experimental study design called the **randomized controlled trial (RCT)**. Here, patients with the disorder are randomly allocated to receive either the experimental treatment or conventional therapy (or a placebo) and then are followed up so that the clinically relevant outcomes of the disease and treatment can be described and compared (see Chapter 3 for more complete details of the RCT design). If you were the woman in our breast cancer example and if, in an improbably objective frame of mind, you wanted to apply epidemiologic principles to determine the treatment of choice, you would want to know if any RCTs had been conducted comparing total mastectomy to more conservative surgery and radiation therapy.

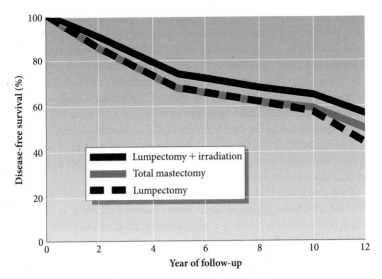

Figure 1-2. Data from a randomized controlled trial showing survival rates after total mastectomy and lumpectomy, with and without irradiation. (From Fisher et al.: Reanalysis and results after 12 years of follow-up in a randomized clinical trial comparing total mastectomy with lumpectomy with or without irradiation in the treatment of breast cancer, N Engl J Med 333:1456–1461, 1995.)

As it turns out, there are several such trials. A recent study found that lumpectomy, with or without irradiation, was equivalent to total mastectomy (Figure 1-2). Similar numbers of women remained disease-free and were alive 12 years after the procedure. So your literature search would give you the ammunition to say that the lumpectomy is less disfiguring than mastectomy and leads to a similar outcome.

How to Identify Health Service Use Needs and Trends

Modern epidemiology plays an important role in the development of methods that can be used to describe health services and to test alternative ways to "deliver the goods." For example, one often-debated health service question concerns the effect of health insurance coverage on the health services used by poor and near-poor populations. Conservatives claim that allowing people free access to health care services will open the floodgates and result in massive increases in health care costs. In so doing, they ignore two kinds of data: (1) the several decades of experience in Canada and western Europe that provide ample demonstration that there is a practical ceiling on use of health services and (2) the unpleasant experience of cooling one's heels in a physician's waiting room, thumbing 10-year-old copies of *Reader's Digest*. The idea that people would prefer this to doing almost anything else is bizarre. By contrast, socialists live in their own version of Utopia where all are equal—in access, income, and reason. In socialist heaven, no clear-thinking individual would dare to take undue advantage of free health care services, and rates of use would not differ regardless of the method of payment.

Obviously, truth lies somewhere in between these extremes. Taube and Rupp conducted a study to assess the effect of Medicaid coverage on access to ambulatory mental health care for the poor and near-poor less than 65 years of age. By analyzing data from the National Medical Care Utilization and Expenditure Survey, they found that the poor and near-poor with continuous Medicaid coverage used almost twice as much service as the poor and near-poor not enrolled in Medicaid (Figure 1-3).

They concluded that the higher probability of use in those covered by Medicaid reflects the impact of the increased financial accessibility to needed mental health services. (This is a fine demonstration of the art of science-manship. Take an obvious and self-evident conclusion from the data, and clothe it in big obscure words so it sounds profound.)

This is only one example. Our personal favorite, which neatly skewers those who assume that every additional dollar spent on health care is a dollar well spent, is the repeated demonstration (in Scandinavia, Israel, and Canada) that when the physicians go on a protracted strike, the mortality rate drops.

Some other variations on this theme are *health economics*, which combines epidemiologic and economic methods to examine the cost-effectiveness of alternative models of delivery, and *policy analysis*, which seeks to link research findings to change in health policy.

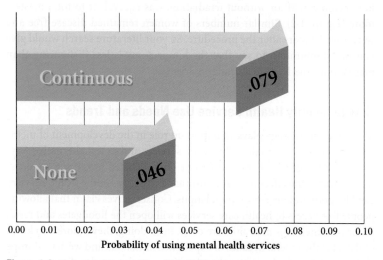

Figure 1-3. Data showing the effect of Medicaid coverage on access to ambulatory mental health care for the poor and near-poor populations less than 65 years of age. (From Taube CA, Rupp A: The effect of Medicaid on access to ambulatory mental health care for the poor and near-poor, Med Care 24:677–687, 1986.)

A DOSE OF REALITY

So far, epidemiology has been presented as if it's the answer to life, the universe, and everything, and indeed, some true believers actually feel this way. But, before we venture into this brave new world, it's worthwhile pointing out some of its limitations.

Epidemiology, and the related field of population health, has the potential for looking at disease in a broader, more holistic way, taking into account not only germs and our genetic predispositions, but also psychological factors such as stress and social support; and sociocultural ones like poverty, access to care, and gender and racial disparities in disorders such as hypertension, diabetes, and cancer. However, there is a countervailing tendency to reduce all of these factors into what McKinlay and Marceau call "biophysiologic reductionism"; an attempt to explain them in terms of biology and physiology. For example, the **Whitehall II study** (which we'll mention again in Chapter 3) found that the lowest-ranking British civil servants had mortality and morbidity rates three times higher than those in the top echelon. One proposed explanation, the **Barker hypothesis**, holds that biological predispositions are set *in utero*, so that those in the lowest social classes are destined to become ill because of their mothers' behaviors (e.g., smoking, poor nutrition) and genetics. Although obviously variables such as these are important, reductionism has the unfortunate effect of narrowing the focus of research and intervention to only those factors for which biological links can be established and ameliorated, and away from broader, more social and cultural ones.

Perhaps related to this, we are still plagued (to use an epidemiological term) with thinking that health and disease are two different states, rather than points along a continuum. We try to cram our data into 2×2 tables, with the outcome being improved versus not improved, alive or dead, with the disease or without the disease, and so on. This may simplify our statistics, but it doesn't correspond to reality. With most conditions, it makes more sense to ask "How much of the disease does the person have?" rather than "Is it present or not?" For example, there isn't a clear dividing line between having and not having cancer. At what point cellular abnormalities and dysplasias become large enough to be considered cancerous is a definitional issue, drawing what is often an artificial line in the sand. This, too, constrains our thinking regarding both mechanisms and interventions.

Another limitation of epidemiology pointed out by McKinlay and Marceau is the fact that most of it is totally atheoretical. Much of what passes for clinical epidemiology is little more than technology assessment—what happens if we give drug A through orifice M to patients with disease Y?—without much thought to why A, M, or Y. Indeed, some in the field have advocated using what statisticians call "one-tailed tests"—looking only at whether intervention A is better than treatment B, and not being concerned if it is worse. From our perspective, this is not science; a scientist would want to know *why* his or her theory went wrong so that it could be modified and improved. For example, beta carotene was seen as a natural anti-cancer agent, but two trials were stopped because in one, those taking it had 28% *more* lung cancer than controls. A one-tailed test would have led to dismissal of these findings as chance; perhaps a good evaluation of the technology, but terrible for our understanding. Because of the unexpected results, we now understand more about the effects of beta carotene on the cellular structure of the lungs. Too much epidemiology is what Smith (1985) describes as "a vast stock-pile of almost surgically clean data untouched by human thought." Without theory to guide our research, we may stumble on findings, but the field as a whole will progress only fitfully.

It is more than a simple question of what statistical test to use. Giacomini recently wrote an article criticizing the considerable research on "intercessionary prayer," wherein people with a disease are randomized, without their knowledge, to one group where parishioners of various denominations pray for them ("intercedes with prayer") or another group which does without, then they see who lives longer. Study of intercessionary prayer has a long history, dating back to Francis Galton in the late 1800s, as we will describe later. Recent history, however, is that after four million dollars and many trials, the results have been inconclusive (except for one tongue in cheek trial reported in BMJ, where the prayer was done retroactively, after the patients had died. Regrettably, this has been included as an exemplary study in several systematic reviews). Giacomini's point is not that the studies were poorly done; in fact, the methodological quality was generally good. Her thesis is that the trials make no sense because there is no credible scientific theory underlying the intervention. Either it is based on belief in God, which cannot be scientifically proven or standardized, or on some physical mode of transmission. In the latter case, despite appeals to collapsed wave functions or quantum states, there is no credible physical mechanism that would apply uniquely to the sending and receiving of prayer. Thus, the question is not scientifically credible, for want of a good theory, not for poor methods.

Possibly because of inattention to theory, we are constantly confusing physiological and biological factors that may simply indicate that a disease is present with ones that actually cause the disease. That is, we misinterpret *markers* of a disorder with *causes* of it. As we point out in the next chapter, this has led to some spectacular failures—drugs that lower "bad" cholesterol levels but do nothing for reducing mortality; or ones that lower plaque levels in the brain but don't affect the symptoms of Alzheimer's disease. Compounding the problem, the results from large epidemiological surveys that try to uncover the causes of illness have had mixed results. We documented some successes earlier in this chapter, to which we can add the relationship between smoking and lung cancer, asbestos and mesothelioma, hypertension and heart failure, exposure to sunlight and skin cancer, and others. But, there have also been colossal blunders. The Nurses' Health Study found in 1985 that women taking estrogen had only one-third the number of heart attacks as those who did not take it, resulting in hormone replacement therapy becoming standard practice. Thirteen years later, the Heart and Estrogen-progestin Replacement Study (HERS), and then the Women's Health Initiative (WHI) concluded that estrogen actually put women at *greater* risk of heart disease, stroke, and other problems. And now we've flipped yet again and declared that it *should* be used by women in early menopause. Other examples, where RCTs later disproved the "effectiveness" of interventions seen with observational studies include beta-carotene, and vitamins C and E for cardiovascular disease, and fiber for colon cancer. The list goes on, but we'll stop here. Of course, we should remind the reader that, despite some pronouncements from avid trialists, the solution to bad theory is not good study design (i.e., the RCT). There are probably as many incidents where the trials disagree among themselves (estrogen being the latest casualty) as where trials and observational studies lead to different conclusions. If it weren't so, we wouldn't need systematic reviews, after all.

We also fail to realize that in health care, as in engineering, things "bite back," and we constantly run into the law of unintended consequences. Have we significantly decreased the mortality rate of people with Down syndrome? Congratulations—we now have a large cohort of people with both Down syndrome and early-onset dementia. The very first RCT was with sulfanilamide, significantly reducing the fatality rate from pneumonia. But, the great 19th century physician, William Osler, correctly called pneumonia "the old man's friend," so we now have more people with Alzheimer's disease living to ripe old ages. Radiation therapy has greatly reduced the mortality in children from leukemia and other cancers, but the treatment also results in cataracts, heart disease, learning disabilities, a 10-fold increase in the probability of future cancers, and perhaps mental retardation. These can be seen as what Gruenberg calls "the failures of success." Focusing on short-term gains blinds us to the long-term consequences of our interventions.

Finally, McKinlay and Marceau mention "dogmatism by design"—the belief that only findings from some research designs (in particular, the RCT) are worthy of belief, and that all other designs are fatally flawed. In fact, we had one student who had difficulty designing a study to measure the retest reliability of a scale because it wouldn't involve a randomized trial. A good research design is one that answers the question, not one that follows a fixed methodology. If you can come up with a randomized controlled trial that examines the effects of second-hand smoke on children's lung functioning, please let us know.

So, welcome to this world of epidemiology. It can tell us a lot about the world, but it cannot answer every question or resolve every issue. Knowing its limitations is as important as learning its strengths.

SUMMARY

Epidemiology is a combination of knowledge and research methods concerned with the distribution and determinants of health and illness in populations and with contributors to health and control of health problems. It comprises an analytic, descriptive component termed *classical epidemiology* and a component concerned with critical appraisal of the research literature and diagnosis and management of illness, which is termed *clinical epidemiology*.

Modern epidemiology contributes to defining new clinical syndromes and their causes and to completing the picture of the natural history and clinical course of a disease. It assists in the identification of the health risks associated with particular exposures and suggests strategies for disease prevention. It provides the criteria and methodology for determining whether a treatment is effective and for describing and identifying health services needs and trends. Epidemiology has application to a range of health-related disciplines and has benefited from the contributions of a variety of professions.

REFERENCES

Alderson M: *An introduction to epidemiology*, ed 2, London, 1983, Macmillan Press.

Cassel JC: Community diagnosis. In Omran AR, editor: *Community medicine in developing countries*, New York, 1974, Springer.

Last JM: *A dictionary of epidemiology*, Oxford, 1983, Oxford University Press.

MacMahon B, Pugh TF: *Epidemiology: principles and methods*, Boston, 1970, Little, Brown.

McFarlane AH, Neale KA, Norman GR: Methodological issues in developing a scale to measure social support, *Schizophr Bull* 7:90–100, 1981.

Norman GR, McFarlane AH, Streiner DL: Health diaries: strategies for compliance and relation to other measures, *Med Care* 20:623–629, 1982.

Oxford English Dictionary, London, 1971, Oxford University Press.

Trends in Epidemiology

Grimes DA, Schulz KF: Descriptive studies: what they can and cannot do, *The Lancet* 359: 145-149, 2002.

McKeown T: *The modern rise of population*, London, 1976, Edward Arnold.

Omran AR: Changing patterns of health and disease during the process of national development. In Omran AR, editor: *Community medicine in developing countries*, New York, 1974, Springer.

Current Applications of Epidemiology

Morris JN: *Uses of epidemiology,* New York, 1975, Churchill Livingstone.

Sackett DL, Haynes RB, Tugwell P: *Clinical epidemiology: a basic science for clinical medicine,* Toronto, 1985, Little, Brown.

Toxic Shock Syndrome

Bergdoll MS, Chesney PJ: *Toxic shock syndrome,* Boca Raton, 1991, CRC Press.

Centers for Disease Control and Prevention: Reduced incidence of menstrual toxic-shock syndrome—United States, 1980–1990, *MMWR* 39:421–423, 1990.

Helgerson SD, Foster LR: Toxic shock syndrome in Oregon: epidemiologic findings, *Ann Intern Med* 96(2):909–911, 1982.

Langmuir AD: Toxic shock syndrome—an epidemiologist's view, *J Infect Dis* 4:588–591, 1992.

Schlech WF, Shands KN, Reingold AL: Risk factors for development of toxic shock syndrome: association with a tampon brand, *JAMA* 7:835–839, 1982.

Stallones RA: A review of the epidemiological studies of toxic shock syndrome, *Ann Intern Med* 96(2):917–920, 1982.

Nuclear "Accidents"

Ahearne J: Nuclear power after Chernobyl, *Science* 236:673–679, 1987.

Bennett B, Repacholi M, Carr Z: Health effects of the Chernobyl accident and special health care programmes. Geneva, 2006, World Health Organization.

Baverstock KF: A preliminary assessment of the consequences for inhabitants of the UK of the Chernobyl accident, *Int J Radiat Biol* 50:3–13, 1986.

Fernberg SE, Bromet EJ, Follman D: Longitudinal analysis of categorical epidemiological data: a study of Three Mile Island, *Environ Health Perspect* 63:241–248, 1985.

Mettler FA, Williamson MR, Henry D: Thyroid nodules in the population living around Chernobyl, *JAMA* 268:616–619,1992.

Parkin DM, Cardis E, Masuyer E: Childhood leukemia following the Chernobyl accident: the European Childhood Leukemia-Lymphoma Incidence Study, *Eur J Cancer* 29A:87–95, 1993.

Urea Formaldehyde Foam Insulation

Norman GR, Newhouse MT: Health effects of ureaformaldehyde foam insulation: evidence of causation, *Can Med Assoc J* 134:733–737, 1986.

Strategies for Prevention

Munroe Blum H, Boyle MH, Offord DR: Single-parent families—child psychiatric disorder and school performance, *J Am Acad Child Adolesc Psychiatry* 27:214–219, 1988.

Offord DR: Prevention of behavioral and emotional disorders in children, *J Child Psychol Psychiatry* 29:9–19, 1987.

Treatment of Early Breast Cancer

Fisher B, Anderson S, Redmond CK: Reanalysis and results after 12 years of follow-up in a randomized clinical trial comparing total mastectomy with lumpectomy with or without irradiation in the treatment of breast cancer, *N Engl J Med* 333:1456–1461, 1995.

Health Insurance Coverage

Taube CA, Rupp A: The effect of Medicaid on access to ambulatory mental health care for the poor and near-poor, *Med Care* 24:677–687, 1986.

A Dose of Reality

Barker D: *Mothers, babies and disease in later life*, London, 1994, BMJ Publications.

DeLaat CA, Lampkin BC: Long-term survivors of childhood cancer: evaluation and identification of sequelae of treatment, *CA* 42:263–282, 1992.

Giacomini M (in press): Theory-based medicine and the role of evidence: why the emperor needs new clothes, again. *Perspect Biol Med*.

Gruenberg EM: The failures of success. *Milbank Mem Fund Q* 55:3–24, 1977.

Hsia J, Langer RD, Manson JE, et al.: Conjugated equine estrogens and coronary heart disease: the Women's Health Initiative, *Arch Intern Med* 166:357–365, 2006.

Hulley S, Grady D, Bush T, et al.: Randomized trial of estrogen plus progestin for secondary prevention of coronary heart disease in postmenopausal women. Heart and Estrogen/progestin Replacement Study (HERS) Research Group. *JAMA* 280:605–613, 1998.

Marmot MG, Smith GD, Stansfeld S, et al.: Health inequalities among British civil servants: the Whitehall II study, *The Lancet* 337:1387–93, 1991.

McKinlay JB, Marceau LD: To boldly go . . . *Am J Pub Health* 90:25–33, 2000.

Omenn GS, Goodman GE, Thornquist MD, et al.: Effects of a combination of beta carotene and vitamin A on lung cancer and cardiovascular disease. *N Engl J Med* 334:1150–1155, 1996.

Smith A: The epidemiological basis of community medicine. In Smith A, editor: *Recent advances in community medicine 3*, Edinburgh, 1985, Churchill Livingstone.

Smith GD, Ebrahim S: Epidemiology—is it time to call it a day? *Int J Epidemiol* 30:1–11, 2001.

Stampfer MJ, Willett WC, Colditz GA, et al.: A prospective study of postmenopausal estrogen therapy and coronary heart disease, *N Engl J Med* 313:1044–1049, 1985.

Tenner E: *Why things bite back: Technology and the revenge of unintended consequences*, New York, 1996, Vintage Books.

TO READ FURTHER

Fletcher RH, Fletcher SW, Wagner EH: *Clinical epidemiology: the essentials*, Baltimore, 1982, Williams & Wilkins.

Henneckens CH, Buring JE: *Epidemiology in medicine*, Boston, 1987, Little, Brown.

MacMahon B, Pugh TF: *Epidemiology: principles and methods*, Boston, 1970, Little, Brown.

Omran AR: Changing patterns of health and disease during the process of national development. In Omran AR, editor: *Community medicine in developing countries,* New York, 1974, Springer.

Sackett DL, Haynes RB, Tugwell P: *Clinical epidemiology: a basic science for clinical medicine,* Toronto, 1985, Little, Brown.

Classical Epidemiology

A LITTLE BIT OF HISTORY

As we mentioned in Chapter 1, classical, or big-E, epidemiology is concerned with description and hypothesis testing of groups of people. As with most things in medicine, we can find the early roots of classical epidemiology in the Bible and in the works of Hippocrates, especially if we squint a bit and don't take what's written too literally. In fact some of the parallels between biblical and contemporary experience are remarkable.

The first census is detailed, appropriately enough, in the fourth book of the Bible, *Numbers*. Today it would be labeled as sexist (it counted only men), ageist (it counted only men more than 20 years of age), and militaristic (its purpose was to count potential warriors). Also presaging recent events, there are still fierce battles about its accuracy, although the allegations are of overcounting (by a factor of 10) rather than undercounting. *Numbers* resembles modern books of statistics in other ways: it consists of long lists of facts, it is incredibly boring to read, and it contains much data but little in the way of knowledge.

A later census was ordered by King David, which took almost 10 months to complete. Given the size of the population they were dealing with, this actually makes our modern bureaucrats look efficient, especially because the Israelites weren't also concerned with counting the number of indoor toilets or TV sets. Corresponding to many contemporary beliefs, *Chronicles* states that David was told to do this by Satan, and as a result many plagues were visited upon the Israelites. In fact the Old Testament is replete with plagues. As anyone who has ever attended a Passover Seder knows, the Egyptians alone were smitten with 10 of them, ranging from boils to locusts, just to convince them to let the Israelites go. Unfortunately, the descriptions of many of the plagues leave us wondering just what it was that the people of biblical times had. For example, leprosy is mentioned in a number of places, but it covers a multitude of skin disorders, only some of which are contagious and chronic. Other plagues leave more room for speculative translation of the type that does not find its way into Sabbath sermons (at least none that we've attended). For instance, there is a phrase in Deuteronomy that states, "The Lord will smite thee with the botch of Egypt and with *ophalim* and with *garab* and with *cheres*, from which thou canst not be healed." Various scholars have translated *ophalim* to mean hemorrhoids, venereal ulcers, or even venereal prolapse, none of which will kill you, but which are still things you wouldn't want to tell your mother about or have for the rest of your life.

The Hippocratic writings are voluminous and contain among them books called *Epidemics* and *Air, Water, Places*. Because it was then believed that all diseases were caused by imbalances among the four humors (i.e., blood, phlegm, black bile, and yellow bile; not Richard Pryor, Jackie Mason, Bob Newhart, and Mort Sahl), it was felt that the physician had to know when humors exert their influence, what diseases they cause in each season, and what their manifestations are. Also, regions differ in terms of their temperature, humidity, and openness to winds, all of which were felt to influence the health of people. Thus the physician had to be aware of the environment and its effects on illness and well-being, factors that are considered today even by humorless epidemiologists.

Not much happened (at least as far as we're concerned) until the end of the seventeenth century when John Graunt wrote *Natural and Political Observations Made upon the Bills of Mortality*. Based on Bills of Mortality (what we would today call death records) he gathered from parishes in London and Hampshire, Graunt attempted to draw some conclusions about matters of life and death. He discovered, for example, that (1) there were a larger number of boys born than girls, (2) the mortality rate increased in the autumn ("the most unhealthfull season"), and (3) "some *Diseases*, and *Casualties* keep a constant proportion, whereas some others are very irregular." By looking at changes over time, Graunt was able to identify diseases that increased in mortality (e.g., rickets and "a stopping of the stomach"), stayed the same ("the gout"), or even decreased ("the stones"). One of his most insightful observations is shown in Figure 2-1, depicting the survival rate as a function of age. (He reported this in a table because Descartes was only then inventing graphs.) None of these findings would strike us as revolutionary today, but at the time they reflected a major shift in thinking: individual reports can be summarized to draw general conclusions, and there are natural laws that govern patterns of birth and death. Also, some of his "positions" are as germane today as they were in 1662 when his book was published: "The ignorance of the *Searchers* [should be] no impediment to the keeping of sufficient, and useful Accompts," and that "A true Accompt of the *Plague* cannot be kept, without the Accompt of other *Diseases*." Another position illustrates either the fragility of men or the beneficial effect of medical care: "*Physicians* have two *Women* Patients to one *Man*, and yet more Men die then [sic] Women."

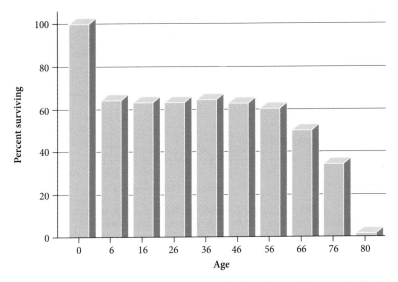

Figure 2-1. Survival rate as a function of age. (Modified from Graunt J: Natural and political observations made upon the Bills of Mortality, Baltimore, 1939, Johns Hopkins Press.)

Again, things were pretty quiet, epidemiologically speaking, for approximately 150 years. Then within a few years of each other, there were two studies of infectious diseases that laid the foundation for classical epidemiology and used methods that are still part of our armamentarium. In 1846 there was an outbreak of measles in the Danish Faroe Islands. The physician who investigated the epidemic, Peter Ludwig Panum, determined (1) that there is a delay between the time of exposure and the development of the rash (**incubation period**), (2) that the disease is transmitted by direct contact between infected and susceptible people and does not arise spontaneously or because of "miasma," (3) when people with the disease were infectious, and (4) most importantly, that a previous bout of measles protected people from subsequent attacks.

Approximately 10 years later, John Snow investigated the causes of the increased rates of cholera in certain areas of London. He observed that the disease was most prevalent in districts supplied with water by the Lambeth Company and the Southwark and Vauxhall Company, both of which obtained their water from a section of the Thames River that was extremely polluted with sewage. He also noted that the rate of new cases of cholera declined in those households supplied by the Lambeth Company after it relocated its intake pipe to a less polluted part of the Thames River. At the same time, there was no change in the incidence of the disease in homes supplied by the Southwark and Vauxhall Company, which continued to draw its water from the heavily polluted section of the river (Figure 2-2). Making this an even better "experiment of nature," the water supply pipes

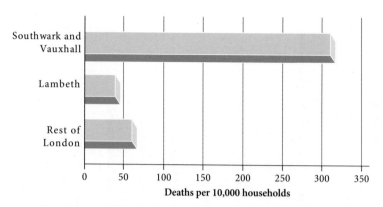

Figure 2-2. Deaths from cholera in houses supplied by two different water companies in London. (Modified from Snow J: On the mode of communication of cholera, ed 2, London, 1855, Churchill. [Reprinted in Snow on cholera, New York, 1936, Commonwealth Fund.])

to the individual houses had remained where they were, so adjacent houses were often supplied by the two different companies.

Snow's brilliance lay in his recognition of the opportunity to test his hypothesis, which was that drinking water from the Southwark and Vauxhall Company increased the risk of cholera compared with the water supplied by the Lambeth Company. In his book, *On the Mode of Communication of Cholera*, Snow noted that

> Each company supplies both rich and poor, both large houses and small; there is no difference either in the condition or the occupation of the persons receiving the water of the different companies . . . . The [natural] experiment, too, was on the grandest scale. No fewer than three hundred thousand people of both sexes, of every age and occupation, and of every rank and station, from gentle folks down to the very poor, were divided into two groups without their choice and, in most cases, without their knowledge; one group being supplied with water containing the sewage of London and amongst it, whatever might have come from the cholera patients, the other group having water quite free from such impurity. To turn this grand experiment to account, all that was required was to learn the supply of water to each individual house where a fatal attack of cholera might occur.

Walking from door to door (whoever said that epidemiology is an armchair profession?), Snow documented the source of drinking water for every house where a death from cholera had taken place. In this way, he determined that the polluted water, supplied by the Southwark and Vauxhall Company, was indeed responsible for the cholera epidemic. Snow obviously understood the importance of the two groups being similar in terms of possible confounding factors (a term we will return to in more depth in the next chapter)—variables such as age, housing conditions, socioeconomic status, and gender—which could account for the difference in cholera rates, as opposed to the source of the water. In the remainder of this chapter, we will take a closer look at some of the factors that affect the spread of disease.

The middle of the 19th century—in particular, the Crimean War—brought two other advances to the field, both by the same person. Bloody as that conflict was, 10 times as many people died from communicable diseases such as typhus, typhoid fever, amebic dysentery, and cholera as from battle wounds. Florence Nightingale, "The Lady with the Lamp," is best remembered as the nurse who cleaned up the Scutari base Army hospital, dramatically improving the survival rate of the patients from 57% to 97%. In actuality, she didn't; she brought attention to the problem, but it was the Palmerston Commission that (literally) did the dirty work. What she is less remembered for (or perhaps even despised for by some) is that she was one of the first to use statistical methods to document what was happening. (Remember Graunt? Well, neither did anyone else.) She plotted the incidence of preventable deaths from various causes, along the way inventing new graphical techniques, such as the *polar-area diagram.*

But, we cannot leave the history of epidemiology without mentioning the famous observational studies by Sir Francis Galton in the 1870s. Prevented from doing an intervention trial to study the efficacy of prayer by having clergy pray for patients in one wing of the hospital but not another, he did some secondary data analyses. He reasoned that the most prayed for people in England were the kings and the children of clergymen, so if intercessory prayer worked, they should live longer than lords and children of other professionals (the comparison groups); their lives were slightly shorter. Similarly, ships filled with missionaries sank with a slightly greater frequency and loss of life than other ships. Thus, he concluded, prayer probably didn't have too harmful an effect.

SOME BASIC CONCEPTS

Perhaps the worst epidemic to ever inflict humanity (with the possible exception of purple Barney toys) was the outbreak of bubonic plague, or the black death, that swept through Europe in the middle of the 14th century. Although precise figures on the number of deaths are almost impossible to determine, it has been estimated that one-quarter to one-third of the population of Europe, or 15 million to 20 million people, died. Yet as terrible as these figures are, two points are readily apparent.

First, not everyone was affected. Even in Florence, Italy, the death rate was nearly 70%, but of course 30% of the populace was unaffected. Second, the plague was not always present. It came in waves during a period of a few years, disappearing in the winter and reappearing in the spring, until it finally faded from the scene. The question this raises is why—why some people and not others, why in 1347 and not the previous year, why in the warm months but not winter, why humans and not dogs, and on and on.

Let's take a look at some of the factors that might provide an explanation for some of these questions by using the plague and other disorders as models. Authors tend to group the factors into triads—person, place, and time or agent, host, and environment. "Place" though is just another name for "environment," and "host" is a fancy term for "person" (because we're not discussing animal epidemiology in this book). So after eliminating duplications, we are left with a tradition-breaking tetrad: **agent**, **person**, **place**, and **time**.

Agent

It seems as if every time we open the newspaper, we're greeted with news that something else is going to kill us: if we stay at home, it will be radon gas from the basement or *Cryptosporidium* from the drinking water; if we go out, it will be the cholesterol in the popcorn at the movies or hemolytic uremic syndrome from *E. coli* when we eat at the local hamburger joint. Yet a moment's reflection will tell us that, despite the tenor of these stories, not everything is deadly or even dangerous (otherwise, we wouldn't be here to write this book or you to read it). There are only certain things that are necessary etiologic factors for diseases—what epidemiologists call **agents**. Lilienfeld groups agents into four categories: (1) nutritive, (2) chemical, (3) physical, and (4) infectious.

Some **nutritive agents** can cause disease by an excess of them and others by a deficiency. Too much cholesterol, for example, may lead to coronary heart disease; too much salt may lead to hypertension; too much calcium may lead to kidney stones. On the other hand, too little calcium can lead to osteoporosis (how's that for a bind?); beriberi can result from too little thiamine (vitamin B_1); pellagra can result from too little niacin; kwashiorkor can result from a protein deficiency. **Chemical agents** may consist of allergens (e.g., ragweed, various food dyes, bee venom) or poisons (e.g., arsenic, carbon monoxide, overdoses of heroin or tricyclic antidepressants). Ionizing radiation or ultraviolet light would be considered among the **physical agents** that can lead to problems. Perhaps the most well-known agents to health workers are the **infectious agents**, such as viruses (mumps, measles, Ebola virus, and acquired immunodeficiency syndrome [AIDS]), bacteria (tuberculosis [TB], rheumatic fever, syphilis), protozoa (malaria), or rickettsia (typhus, Rocky Mountain spotted fever).

Person

Agents are necessary to cause disease, but they are not sufficient. Not everyone who is stung by a bee develops an anaphylactic reaction, and two people may enjoy the same meal in Mexico City, but only one may spend the rest of the evening enthroned upon that porcelain perch. It is obvious that people differ in terms of their susceptibility or response to the agents—what are called the **person** or **host factors**.

There are some person characteristics that we are **born with**, like gender (what we used to call "sex"), year of birth, religion, and genetic make-up. For example, there are conditions that occur with a greater frequency within one ethnic group rather than another (e.g., sickle cell anemia among African-Americans, Tay-Sachs disease among Jews from central Europe, thalassemia among Greeks and Italians), or more in one sex than the other (e.g., hemophilia), suggesting a genetic component. Year of birth is somewhat different from age, although the two are obviously related. If I am 50 years old this year (OK, so I shaved off a few years), and you are 30 years old, then in 20 years you will be the same age I am now and susceptible to the same aches and pains. However, what can never change is that you belong to a different **birth cohort**. Figure 2-3 shows the death rate per 100,000 men at different ages (the X-axis) among three cohorts: men born in the decades 1885 to 1894, 1895 to 1904, and 1905 to 1914. The graph indicates that for a man between the ages of 15 and 24 who was born between 1885 and 1894, the death rate was 539.2 per 100,000 men, whereas for someone the same age but born between 1905 and 1914, the death rate was 349.3 per 100,000. Thus although their ages are the same, what they experience is determined in part by when they were born.

Other host factors are **modified** or **acquired with time**, such as age itself and immunologic experience, whether achieved naturally through prior exposure (as occurred with some people in Panum's study of measles) or artificially through inoculation. Chronic illnesses, such as emphysema, which increase a person's susceptibility to other disorders, would be another example of an acquired host factor. Figure 2-4 shows a condition that although not a disease in the classical sense, is a state that is affected by age. The data, taken from Giambra, show the proportion of people responding "Usually True," "True," or "Very True" to the statement: "Whenever I am bored, I daydream about the opposite sex." The implications of this for one's mental health are best left to those people more than

Figure 2-3. Mortality rates of men at different ages born in various decades. (Data from Spiegelman M, Erhardt CL: Mortality and longevity in the United States. In Erhardt CL, Berlin JE, editors: Mortality and morbidity in the United States, Cambridge, Mass., 1974, Harvard University Press.)

Figure 2-4. % of people of different ages who daydream about the opposite sex when bored. (Data from Giambra LM: Daydreaming across the life span: late adolescent to senior citizen, Int J Aging Hum Dev 5:115–140, 1974.)

45 years of age, who obviously have more time to daydream about these more mundane matters.

Looking at the number of people who acquire a disease at different ages can also suggest hypotheses about etiology. For example, Figure 2-5 shows the incidence of Hodgkin's disease in Brooklyn between 1943 and 1952. Two peaks stand out, one in the late 20s and another much later in life. This has led to speculation that there are two different processes occurring, a biologic agent of low infectivity early on and a mechanism more like that of other lymphomas that affects older people.

A third class of person factors is more **transitory**, like time-limited comorbid conditions, fatigue, or nutritional status. It was likely that factors such as these accounted for varying death rates from the plague from one town to another and why some people survived while others in the same household did not. Finally, some host factors depend on our **behavior**— what yuppies would call *lifestyle*: whether we exercise, how we make use of health services, what we eat, and so on (all of which ignore the famous dictum "Eat well, exercise, still you die").

These categories obviously overlap. Certain behaviors, for instance, have much to do with religion, which for most people is acquired at birth and does not change. Some religions are strictly vegetarian and others prohibit smoking and drinking (those that forbid sex, such as the Shakers, are

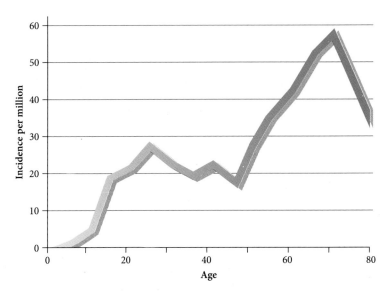

Figure 2-5. Incidence of Hodgkin's disease by age. (Data from MacMahon B: Epidemiological evidence on the nature of Hodgkin's disease, Cancer 10:1045–1054, 1957.)

sort of self-limiting). So look at these more as conceptual guides, rather than fixed differentiations among person variables.

Place

If we look at Figure 2-6, we can see that there is a strong association between the estimated daily fat intake for women in 39 different countries and breast cancer mortality rates, which highlights the role of **place**. It is obvious that place, which is also referred to as **environment**, is rarely a direct factor in its own right. Rather, it reflects a host of other factors that are distributed geographically, including (1) climate (as Hippocrates himself pointed out), (2) diet (as in the case of breast cancer and neural tube defects), (3) cultural practices, (4) methods of food preparation and storage, (5) population density, (6) exposure to pollutants, (7) the presence of arthropods (a fancy name for insects and bugs) that carry disease, and on and on.

The challenge for epidemiologists, once having found differences in the prevalence of some disorder from one place to another, is to discover what it is about the environment that gives rise to these variations. Sometimes this is relatively straightforward. For example, trypanosomiasis occurs only in regions where the tsetse fly lives (if you haven't guessed, that's a fancy name for sleeping sickness). Other relationships require much more ingenuity to uncover. It was known for some time that people living in certain regions of the Far East were at a much higher risk for developing cancers in the

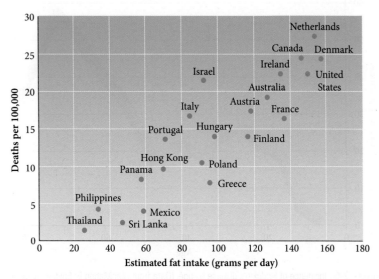

Figure 2-6. Geographic comparisons demonstrate a strong relationship between breast cancer mortality rates and the intake of dietary fat. (Data from Cohen LA: Diet and cancer, Sci Am 257:42–48, 1987.)

gastrointestinal tract than people living elsewhere, even higher than people of Asian descent residing in other countries. This latter would eliminate genetics as a factor, but it would still leave pathogens in the soil, pollutants from nearby factories, diet, or a plethora of other potential agents as contributors. As it turned out, the culprit was diet—specifically, the pickled foods that are considered a delicacy and eaten in relatively large quantities.

Time

Variations in the **time** and occurrence of a particular disease or condition can suggest casual relationships among variables (obviously, this overlaps with year of birth in some cases). As you'll see in Chapter 5, cause and effect cannot be proven simply by finding correlations over time because many other factors are also changing during the interval of which we may or may not be aware; however, as with place, it gives us a place to start looking. For example, in many countries there has been a dramatic decline in the incidence of dental caries during the past 25 years, which started with the gradual introduction of fluoride into community water systems and of fluoride rinsing programs in schools and dentists' offices. Data from New Zealand show that an average 12-year-old in 1971 would have had nine decayed, missing, or filled (DMF) teeth, whereas in 1983 he or she would have had three DMF teeth (Figure 2-7).

This strongly suggests a preventive role for fluoride because no other factors have been introduced or changed simultaneously on such a massive scale that might otherwise explain the decline of tooth decay. This

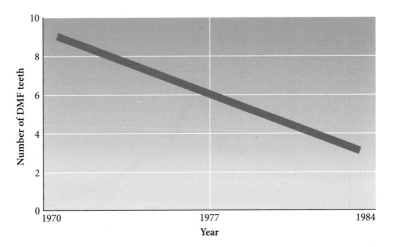

Figure 2-7. Time variable suggests causal relationship between decline in decayed, missing, and filled teeth (DMF) and the use of fluoride in New Zealand.

finding probably also explains why more and more kids and yuppies are wearing braces and having cosmetic dentistry done—dentists have to pay mortgages, too!

The influence of time can also be seen in disorders that occur cyclically or seasonally. We have already discussed the seasonal nature of the black death, which occurred because fleas wanted to escape the cold as much as Canadians. Other disorders that show a cyclical pattern include infectious diseases such as the flu, seasonal affective disorder, and suicide. We might expect suicide to be more prevalent during December or January, when the days are shortest (at least in the northern hemisphere) and the family-oriented holidays exacerbate the loneliness of unattached people, but such is not the case. In fact, as we can see in Figure 2-8, suicides actually peak in June, for reasons that are not fully understood. In this case, the time trend highlights our ignorance of possible causes.

RISK FACTORS

One term that we'll encounter in various guises throughout this book is a **risk factor**. Indeed, we've already run into it in Chapter 1, when we said that one of the aims of epidemiology is assessing the risk associated with harmful exposure. We wisely didn't define the term then, relying on your intuitive understanding of the term. But, as anyone with the slightest knowledge of statistics and epidemiology knows, the way the *cognoscenti* use a term rarely corresponds to common sense; after all, to a statistician, "regression" has nothing to do with thumb-sucking or reverting back to a previous life as a princess in ancient Egypt. (As a totally irrelevant aside,

Figure 2-8. Number of suicides per month per 100,000 people in cities with more than 100,000 inhabitants. (Data from Dublin LI: Suicide: a sociological and statistical study, New York, 1963, Ronald Press.)

have you ever noticed that probably fewer than 0.1% of our ancestors were actually nobles, but that 99.38% of those who claim to have lived previous lives did so as one of the elite?) Well, it's time to bite the bullet and define risk more formally. It seems, though, that the shorter the word or phrase, the more difficult it is to pin down. That's definitely the case with this term. Last, who has written the definitive dictionary in epidemiology, defines a risk factor as:

> An aspect of personal behavior or lifestyle, an environmental exposure, or an inborn or inherited characteristic which on the basis of epidemiological evidence is known to be associated with health-related condition(s) considered important to prevent.

What's interesting about this definition is that it says that a risk factor is *associated* with a health condition; it doesn't say it *causes* it. We know that some risk factors actually are causal, while others may not be, so to try to distinguish among the different usages, various people have talked about different types of risk factors. A **risk determinant** is one that *is* causally related to some outcome—asbestos with mesothelioma, human papillomavirus (HPV) with skin warts, or Canadian politics with terminal boredom (or *ennui* in Quebec).

A **risk marker** is some factor that is associated with a higher probability or prevalence of the outcome, but may not be a cause of it. Being lower down on the economic pecking order is associated with poorer health, but poverty per se is not the culprit. The famous Whitehall I and Whitehall II studies in Great Britain showed that the risk of mortality, especially due to cardiovascular disease (CVD), was inversely related to a person's rank in the civil service. However, even the people at the low end of the scale made a decent living, and health care is universal in England, so something else must be at play. As it turns out, socioeconomic status is actually a marker for other factors, such as smoking, obesity, a sedentary lifestyle, and a lack of control over one's life, that adversely affect health. Finally, a **modifiable risk factor** is a determinant of the outcome than can be altered, changing the risk.

A major problem arises when people mistake a risk marker for a modifiable risk factor. The history of medicine is littered with the remains of studies that tried to modify some putative risk factor, only to find out that it's only a risk marker. For example, it's well known that men are more prone to heart attacks than women, and that this difference disappears after menopause. Aha! Estrogen must be the risk factor, and we can modify that, so let's give it to men. Bad move; the men started dropping like flies. Sadly, there are many other examples: a low-fat diet did nothing to reduce the risk of CVD or breast cancer in women; lowering homocystine concentration did not affect CVD or dementia; and reducing plaque levels in the brain doesn't slow neurodegeneration in patients with Alzheimer's disease. Indeed, there is also some speculation that lowering LDL cholesterol doesn't prevent heart attacks, as witnessed by the early stopping of some trials where drugs that lowered it and raised HDL cholesterol actually resulted in more strokes and heart attacks.

SOME OTHER TERMS YOU SHOULD KNOW

Now that you are becoming somewhat of a maven in the area of classical epidemiology, you should know the precise meaning of a few terms, so let's start with epidemic itself. Traditionally, an **epidemic** refers to the outbreak of a disease in a localized group of people. It can be infectious and spread from one person to another by (1) **carriers** (i.e., people who are susceptible to the disease, although they may not be affected by it themselves, as with Mary for typhoid fever) or (2) **vectors** (intermediate organisms that carry the disease but do not have it, such as the anopheles mosquito for malaria or fleas for the plague). An epidemic can also be caused by the sudden introduction of some pathogen, as happened with Legionnares' disease. Epidemics are usually limited in time, although the time can be long, as we are seeing in the case of AIDS. Sometimes, epidemic is used more broadly, in a social sense. Thus, we hear about "epidemics" of obesity in North America, or epidemics of violence in some parts of Africa. However, this usage is more metaphorical than epidemiological.

In contrast, an **endemic** disease (from the Greek meaning "within the people") is present if cases are localized in one region; for example, river blindness or malaria in certain parts of Africa. When an endemic disease is in a **steady state**, then an affected person infects, on average, one person. We say "on average" because there will always be people who are immune to the disease, so the infected person may actually have to work a bit harder to maintain that average. If fewer people are infected, then the disease will soon die out (as likely happened with the Ebola virus); if more people are infected, then the number of affected people first grows exponentially (i.e., it becomes an **epidemic**), and then reaches a steady state, as it runs out of potential hosts. When an epidemic escapes its local region and starts to affect people over a large portion of the country or even the world, it is said to be **pandemic**. In this regard, the bubonic plague of the 14th century would more properly be called a pandemic rather than an epidemic.

REFERENCES
A Little Bit of History

Galton F: Statistical inquiries into the efficacy of prayer. *Fortnight Rev* 12:125–136, 1874.
Graunt J: *Natural and political observations made upon the Bills of Mortality*, Baltimore, 1939, Johns Hopkins Press.

Heilig JS: Testing the power of belief [letter]. *Science* 276:881, 1997.

Lilienfeld AM: *Foundations of epidemiology*, New York, 1976, Oxford University Press. Panum PL: *Observations made during the epidemic of measles on the Faroe Islands in the year 1846*, New York, 1940, American Public Health Association.

Phillips ED: *Aspects of Greek medicine*, New York, 1973, St. Martin's Press.

Rosner F, translator: *Julius Preuss' biblical and Talmudic medicine*, New York, 1978, Sanhedrin Press.

Small H: *Florence Nightingale: avenging angel*, New York, 1999, St. Martin's.

Snow J: *On the mode of communication of cholera*, ed 2, London, 1855, Churchill. (Reprinted in *Snow on cholera*, New York, 1936, Commonwealth Fund.)

Some Basic Concepts

Tuchman BW: A *distant mirror*, New York, 1978, Knopf.

Agent

Lilienfeld AM: *Foundations of epidemiology*, New York, 1976, Oxford University Press.

Person

Giambra LM: Daydreaming across the life span: late adolescent to senior citizen, *Int J Aging Hum Dev* 5:115–140, 1974.

Hellman S, Jaffe ES, DeVita Jr VT: Hodgkin's disease. In DeVita Jr VT, Hellman S, Rosenberg SA, editors: *Cancer: principles and practice of oncology*, ed 3, Philadelphia, 1989, Lippincott.

MacMahon B: Epidemiological evidence on the nature of Hodgkin's disease, *Cancer* 10:1045–1054, 1957.

Place

Cohen LA: Diet and cancer, *Sci Am* 257:42–48, 1987.

Time

Dublin LI: *Suicide: a sociological and statistical study*, New York, 1963, Ronald Press.

Spiegelman M, Erhardt CL: Mortality and longevity in the United States. In Erhardt CL, Berlin JE, editors: *Mortality and morbidity in the United States*, Cambridge, Mass., 1974, Harvard University Press.

Working Group on the Federation Dentaire Internationale and the World Health Organization: Changing patterns of oral health and implications for oral health manpower, vol 1, *Int Dent J* 35:235–251, 1985.

RISK FACTORS

Burt BA: Definitions of risk, *J Dent Educ* 65:1007–1008, 2001.

Clarke R, Lewington S, Sherliker P, Armitage J: Effects of B-vitamins on plasma homocystine concentrations and on risk of cardiovascular disease and dementia, *Curr Opin Clin Nutr Metab Care* 10:32–39, 2007.

Coronary Drug Project Research Group: The Coronary Drug Project: findings leading to discontinuation of the 2.5-mg day estrogen group. *JAMA.* 226:652–657, 1973.

Cutler DM: The demise of the blockbuster? *NEJM* 356:1292–1293, 2007.

Holmes C, Boche D, Wilkinson D, Yadegarfar G, Hopkins V, Bayer A, et al.: Long-term effects of $A\beta_{42}$ immunisation in Alzheimer's disease: follow-up of a randomised, placebo-controlled phase I trial, *Lancet* 372:216–223, 2008.

Howard BV, Van Horn L, Hsia, J, Manson, J, Stefanick ML, Wassertheil-Smoller S, et al.: Low-fat dietary pattern and risk of cardiovascular disease: the Women's Health Initiative Randomized Controlled Dietary Modification Trial, *JAMA* 295:655–666, 2006. Last JM: *A dictionary of epidemiology,* ed 4, New York, 2001, Oxford University Press.

Marmot MG, Davey Smith G, Stansfeld SA, Patel C, North F, Head J et al.: Health inequalities among British Civil Servants: the Whitehall II study, *Lancet* 337: 1387–1393, 1991.

Prentice, RL, Caan, B., Chlebowski RT, Patterson R, Kuller LH, Ockene JK, et al.: Low-fat dietary pattern and risk of invasive breast cancer: the Women's Health Initiative Randomized Controlled Dietary Modification Trial, *JAMA* 295: 629–642, 2006.

Taubes G: *Good calories, bad calories: challenging the conventional wisdom on diet, weight control and disease,* New York, 2007, Knopf.

Wadman W: Harsh spotlight falls on Vytorin, *Nat Med* 14:471, 2008.

Research Methodology

In 2000, a neurologist in the U.S. filed a lawsuit for $800 million against Motorola and Verizon, claiming that chronic addiction to his habit of cell phone use led to brain cancer. Then, a 2008 study reported that those who used cell phones regularly had a higher incidence of ipsilateral parotid gland tumors, compared with both irregular users (i.e., people who did not use phones on a regular basis; not those who used them but were constipated) and contralateral tumors. On the other hand, a study of more than 420,000 cell phone users in Denmark did not find any association with brain or salivary gland tumors or leukemia. Cell phones emit nonionizing radiation in the radiofrequency (RF) energy range, and that's what microwave ovens use to heat food. So, what's the story—does cell phone use cook the brain or not? (Anecdotal evidence, gleaned from overhearing teenagers on the phone saying, "And then I go, like, duh," is insufficient, as other evidence confirms the fact that there is no functioning cerebral cortex until a person reaches the age of 29.) Considering that at the current rate of growth, the number of cell phone users will soon exceed the population of the world thrice over, this is an important issue.

The task of the epidemiologist in this situation is twofold: (1) to determine whether there is indeed an increased risk of cancers in the head caused by cell phone use and (2) if so, to determine what the magnitude of that risk is. In this section, we explore some of the possible research designs that could be used to answer these questions. We begin with the basic elements of research design, then discuss various factors, called **threats to validity**, that may lead us to draw erroneous conclusions from the data, and then show how the different design elements can be combined into various types of studies to minimize these threats to validity.

When discussing the different types of sampling strategies, biases, designs, and other elements our aim is not to be comprehensive; any such compendium is always incomplete, because the number of types is based solely on the imagination and inventiveness of the researcher. Rather, we mention some of the more common varieties of each of these factors to illustrate how they can be combined in various ways to address different issues.

YET SOME MORE HISTORY

We like to think that scientific reasoning and research design started with our generation or at least during the Age of Enlightenment. Yet again, though, the Bible beat us to the punch. Before Daniel had his famous encounter with the lions, he faced another challenge. King Nebuchadnez-zar of Babylon ordered the Israelites to eat his food and wine "that they should be nourished." But Daniel, obviously reacting to the lack of objective data supporting the King's claim, made a suggestion that would endear him to vegetarians, teetotalers, and researchers alike. Daniel proposed that the King's servants eat his food for 10 days, and his own men (obviously the experimental group) would eat pulse (a type of legume) and drink water. After 10 days, for the subjects in the experimental group, "their counte-nances appeared fairer, and they were fatter in the flesh, than all the youths that did eat the king's food" (the significance level was not reported, and the possibility of divine intervention cannot be discounted).

Yet again the world had to wait approximately 3000 years for the next experiment. Scurvy was a disorder that first came to people's attention in the 16th century, once sailors were able to make long trips. Its symptoms were so varied, including swelling of the gums, loss of teeth, blotches on the skin, and lethargy, that no cause could be identified. After one disastrous voyage beginning in 1740 and ending in 1744, during which the majority of the crew died from the disease, James Lind conducted a trial aboard the *HMS Salisbury*:

> I took twelve patients in the scurvey. . . . Their cases were as similar as I could have them . . . and had one diet common to all . . . . Two of these were ordered each a quart of cyder a day. Two others took twenty-five gutts of elixir vitriol three times a day, upon an empty stomach; using a gargle strongly acidulated with it for their mouths. Two others took two spoonsful of vinegar three times a day, upon an empty stomach; having their gruels and their other food well acidulated with it, as also the gargle for their mouth. Two of the worst patients . . . were put under a course of sea water. Of this, they drank half a pint every day, and sometimes more or less as it operated by way of a gentle physic. Two others had each two oranges and one lemon given them every day. . . . The two remaining patients took the bigness of a nutmeg three times a day, of an electuary recommended by a hospital-surgeon, made of gar-lic, mustard seed, rad raphan, balsam of Peru, and gum myrrh; using for common drink, barley-water well acidulated with tamarinds; by a decoction of which, with the addition of cremor tartar, they were gen-tly purged three or four times during the course.

The two men eating oranges and lemons recuperated completely after a week; the others barely survived their "treatment." This story teaches us two lessons. The first is the power of a good research design (although today, no granting agency would approve a project where the sample size in each group is two). The second is the reaction of bureaucracies. The British Navy, hearing of a cure for a widespread and potentially fatal disorder, did nothing for 42 years. Then it substituted limes, which have far less antiscorbutic properties than lemons but were grown in British territories, whereas lemons had to be imported. The only positive feature of this debacle is that, had lemons been used, Britons would be called Lemonies by Americans rather than Limeys.

But experimental medicine, or what we would now call **clinical epidemiology**, really took off once the *germ theory* of disease became established. Although some of the old timers, such as Avicenna (ca. 1020) and Fracastoro (1546), postulated that diseases such as TB and the plague were transmitted from person to person by invisible, seed-like entities, these remained one untested theory among many others (although Avicenna recommended placing infected people in quarantine—an Italian word meaning 40, which was the number of days for which ships with sick people had to sit in the harbor before passengers could come ashore). In 1653, though, Anton van Leeuwenhoek perfected the microscope, with which he saw *animalcules*, or single-cell organisms. For this, he has been called the "father of microbiology," although as with many other paternity suits, especially in Hollywood, other people have come forward to claim the baby.

In the late 1700s, Edward Jenner noticed that milkmaids did not contract smallpox, a disease which at that time killed about 20% of the population. Suspecting that they were protected by their exposure to the less virulent cowpox, he inoculated a local boy with the pus from a cowpox lesion, and a week later, with smallpox itself. Fortunately for Jenner, medical science, and especially the boy, the kid did not contract the disease. Later, in an experiment that would have a tough time passing muster with today's ethics boards, he did the same thing with a number of children living in an orphanage, with similar results. He called his technique *vaccination*, based on the Latin *vaccinia*, which means cowpox. (This may also be one of the earliest examples of scientific plagiarism. Voltaire noted that Circassian women deliberately gave smallpox to infants "from time immemorial.") In one of the earliest randomized controlled trials after Lind, Louis Pasteur inoculated 25 sheep against anthrax, leaving another 25 as a control group, and all were injected with anthrax (the history books are silent regarding whether the sheep gave signed consent). At the end of the week, all of the inoculated sheep were frolicking around, and the control animals were all dead. Results of our studies should look so good.

Epidemiology remained primarily a medical occupation until the middle of the 19th century, when social scientists invaded the realm (as is their wont). Mental illness was deemed to have its cause in the poverty, anomie, and crowdedness of the big cities, and this emphasis on social factors has influenced almost every major survey in the area ever since. Although the influence of socioeconomic factors has been examined in terms of death rates since roughly the same time (e.g., Chadwick's *Report on an Enquiry into the Sanitary Conditions of the Labouring Population in Great Britain*, in 1842), their role in medical disorders was largely ignored until the famous **Whitehall Studies** and the **Black Report** from England. Not only was there a gradient of morbidity, mortality, and health service use that exactly paralleled the gradient of social class, but this also existed *within* the civil service. Even though all of the participants in the Whitehall Studies were employed and enjoyed (or suffered from) the free medical care of the National Health Service, doorkeepers and messengers had three times the mortality rate of administrators. The long-term employment of social scientists was now insured.

DESIGN ELEMENTS

Experimental or Observational Studies

In **experimental** studies, the intervention is under the control of the researcher. For example, the research team may determine (by random allocation) (1) which subjects receive a novel treatment and which ones get traditional (or no) treatment, (2) when an intervention is carried out in a community, or (3) how much of a new drug each patient is given. The aim is to determine how changes in the **independent variable** (the one under the researcher's control) affect some outcome (the **dependent variable**). By controlling the timing or amount of the intervention or which subjects get it and which ones do not, the chances are minimized that other factors outside of the researcher's control could have affected the results.

By contrast, the researcher does not control the intervention in **observational** studies but rather observes the effects of an experiment in nature. It would be both unethical and impractical, for example, to expose some people to cigarette smoke or putative occupational carcinogens deliberately for 20 years to determine their effects. However, by choice or chance, some people have been exposed so it is possible to draw some tentative conclusions based on observation of these subjects and, if possible, control subjects.

Most well-designed studies of a new treatment are experimental in that the research team determines which subjects receive the new drug or intervention and which ones receive traditional treatment or a placebo. Almost all studies that involve exposure to harmful agents or that try to trace the natural history of a disorder are observational. However, these general rules naturally have exceptions. For example, if a place can be found where cell phone use isn't ubiquitous (Outer Mongolia? Lower Slobovia?), it may be possible to give phones to half of the people, chosen randomly, and not give them to the other half. However, this may be difficult to do for practical reasons, and an observational type of study may be more realistic. However, this may be difficult to do because of practical considerations, and an observational type of study may be more realistic. (Needless to say, researchers cannot control which women become pregnant. The last one who tried was hauled up on morality charges.)

Number of Observations

The simplest research design would involve looking at or measuring the outcome only once. In many cases, such as when the outcome is either present or absent or when the *timing* of the outcome is of minor interest, one observation may be all that is necessary. For example, if the question is whether using cell phones results in a higher incidence of brain cancer, we use a tumor registry to see how many people in our sample developed lesions. The outcome is recorded on only a single occasion.

However, if we were interested in the *time course* of an outcome, one observation is not sufficient. To use a different example, Bagby and his colleagues looked at the effects of a new mental health act introduced toward the end of 1978 on the proportion of psychiatric patients who were involuntarily admitted to the hospital (Figure 3-1). The graph shows a dramatic decline in this type of admission after the new, more restrictive legislation.

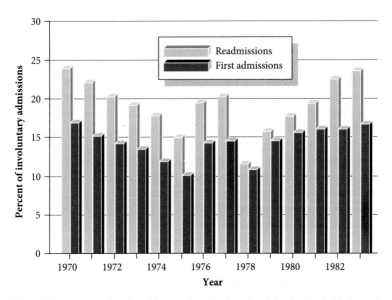

Figure 3-1. The proportion of psychiatric patients involuntarily admitted to hospital before and after the new mental health act of 1978. (From Bagby RM, Silverman I, Ryan DP: Effects of mental health legislative reforms in Ontario, Can Psychol 28:21–29, 1987.)

If the analysis had stopped at this point, it's likely that people would have come to the erroneous conclusion that the new act resulted in a reduction in the proportion of people being admitted to psychiatric wards on an involuntary basis. Multiple observations over time, however, show a different picture, that is, a gradual return to a level even higher than those of the 7 years preceding the new law. So not only do multiple observations tell us something different than a single look, they also reveal something about the "natural history" of the legislation; there was a gradual return to the previous mode of practice as psychiatrists learned to live with the new law.

Direction of Data Gathering

Data can be gathered in one of two ways: (1) looking *forward* and getting new data after the start of the study or (2) looking *backward* and using data that have already been collected. Specific names are used for each of these strategies. Studies that involve gathering data after the study has begun are called **prospective**; in **retrospective** studies, the data have already been recorded for other reasons at some time in the past. The advantage of prospective data collection is that the nature of the data, the definitions of symptoms, the method by which the data are recorded, and other factors can be worked out ahead of time and are constant throughout the course of the trial. In retrospective studies, definitions of symptoms or diseases may have been modified over time, units of measurement may have changed, and old methods for diagnosis may have been replaced, thereby resulting in more variability in the data. Perhaps the greatest advantage of prospective studies is that they allow us to determine the *directionality* of events (i.e., what occurred first and what happened later). As you'll see in Chapter 5, directionality is necessary (but not sufficient) if we want to be able to say anything about causation. Information of this sort is far more difficult (some would say impossible) to obtain accurately in retrospective studies.

Conducting the study retrospectively could involve identifying people who developed brain tumors and then asking them about cell phone use. This has the advantage of being able to be done quickly and cheaply, but it suffers from a number of drawbacks. First, we know that people who have a disorder are more likely to comb their memory to find things they may have done that "caused" it, jeopardizing the accuracy of self-reported behaviors. That means that people with tumors may overestimate how much they used their cell phones. Second, the technology likely would have changed over the years. The RF radiation comes from the antenna, so if there's a gradual shift to hands-free devices, exposure would change over time. A prospective study would enter people into a trial once they started using cell phones (which now means around the age of 18 months). Although the researcher could now record all relevant information with greater accuracy, the study might have to continue for a number of years until enough cases of brain tumors develop.

The term "prospective" should *not* be used to describe trials in which historical data are gathered after a diagnosis or exposure that occurred some time in the past. For example, if we gather hospital utilization data from 1945 to the present on people who witnessed the A-bomb tests in Nevada, the data would still be retrospective, although the hospitalizations occurred after the exposure. Even though the subjects were followed forward in time, the data involve events that happened before *now*; therefore the study would be called "retrospective" (Figure 3-2).

A few authors have tried to clarify this confusion in nomenclature by introducing terms such as "retrolective," "prolective," or "retrospective-prospective." Laudable as this goal is, we feel that these neologisms have only further obfuscated the sufficiently murky picture.

Comparison Groups

Keeping with our study of cell phones and brain tumors, we could easily derive prevalence figures for each of the outcomes of interest (e.g., ipsilateral versus contralateral tumors; those behind the eye and ear, which is near the antenna, versus in other regions of the brain) in a large group of regular cell phone users, but the meaning of the number would be unclear. The major reason is that people who do *not* use cell phones (all seven of them) also experience these adverse effects.

So now the question has become somewhat more complicated: Do people who use cell phones on a regular basis have these outcomes at a *higher rate* than those who don't use cell phones regularly? This means that we

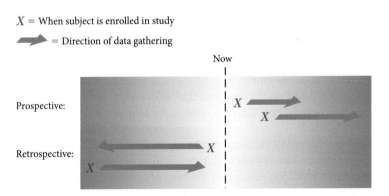

X = When subject is enrolled in study

= Direction of data gathering

Figure 3-2. Prospective versus retrospective studies.

now need a group against which we can compare our prevalence results to determine if the rate is higher.

There are two major types of comparison or control groups: **historical** and **concurrent**. In the former case, we would compare our results with data that already exist from previous studies or tumor registries, making sure that the data were from the pre–cell phone days. If such data do not exist or if they are suspect for one reason or another, the researchers must gather information from a control group concurrently; in essence, there will be at least two groups in the study.

When good historical control groups exist, they can save a considerable amount of time, effort, and expense. Unfortunately, most historical control groups are compromised for one reason or another. The primary reason is that factors in the environment, such a clinical practice, may have changed since the data were originally gathered. For example, advances in diagnostic imaging techniques may allow radiologists to detect tumors that previously would have gone unnoticed, making it seem as if brain cancer were more prevalent now. Also, diagnostic criteria change. This is especially true in psychiatry, in which it seems that every new version of the *Diagnostic and Statistical Manual* classifies the anxiety and eating disorders differently, but we see it in other fields, too. Nodular lymphocyte predominant Hodgkin's lymphoma used to be classified as one of the "classical" Hodgkin's lymphomas, but no longer is, so that prevalence figures will have changed, simply because of the redefinition. The lesson is that when a historical control is used, we have to be certain that nothing has changed in the interim that could affect its comparability with the group we are looking at now.

More commonly, control groups are selected concurrently; that is, at the time that the study is being done. The greatest challenge is selecting a group that does not bias the results one way or the other. For example, if we were looking at the risk factors for contracting MRSA (methicillin-resistant *Staphylococcus aureus*) infection in hospital, we wouldn't want a comparison group made up of people in the community, because they're not at risk for MRSA. Rather, we would chose people who are free of the disease, but are equally at risk—i.e., patients in hospital. The problem is knowing on which variables to match the control subjects with those in the group of interest, and for which variables matching may wipe out true differences (over-matching). Making the issue more problematic, this may change depending on the questions that we're asking. For instance, do we draw the controls from the same unit in the hospital? It all depends. We know that those who have surgical incisions and indwelling catheters are at greater risk of MRSA, so selecting patients from a surgical unit will tell us what factors *over and above* skin penetration put people at greater risk. Conversely, matching patients on the basis of comorbidity precludes finding that this may be a significant risk factor.

It isn't necessary to have one control patient for each case. If the number of cases is small, there may be two, three, or more times the number of controls, simply to increase the sample size. This doesn't bias the results, but after a ratio of about 4:1 controls to cases, the law of diminishing returns kicks in.

On rare occasions a control group may not be necessary at all. To quote Bradford Hill, "If we survey the deaths of infants in the first month of life and find that so many are caused by dropping the baby on its head on the kitchen floor I am not myself convinced that we need controls to satisfy us that this is a bad habit." The classic case of a study where a control group was unnecessary was the use of streptomycin for tuberculous meningitis; without treatment the disease was universally fatal so any improvement in survival was significant. Fortunately or unfortunately, such examples are rare.

Whom to Count

Imagine that we do a study to determine the effects of reading the sister publication of this one, *PDQ Statistics*, on a dread disease first described by us in yet another book, *Biostatistics: The Bare Essentials—photonumerophobia*, which is the fear that our fear of numbers will come to light. Fifty people are given *PDQ* to read, and 50 are given treatment as usual (TAU). At the end of six weeks, we find that two people in the *PDQ* book group haven't read it (bizarre as that may seem) and three have moved out of town, while in the TAU group, four cheated by reading the book, we can't locate one, and one committed suicide. So, whom do we count in the data analysis?

The answer, unsurprisingly, is "It all depends." What it depends on is whether the study is an **efficacy trial** or an **effectiveness trial**. An efficacy study tries to determine whether the treatment *can* work, whereas an effectiveness trial asks if it *does* work. That is, in an efficacy trial, we do everything possible to ensure that we get a positive outcome (short of cheating, that is) if the intervention actually works: we may select only patients who meet rigorous criteria for the disorder, exclude those who have failed on other treatments or who may not adhere to the regimen, call them to remind them to take their meds or to read the book, and so forth. The rationale is that if the intervention doesn't work under these condition, it ain't never going to work. But, in real life, we know that patients don't always comply, those in the control group may deliberately or inadvertently get the active treatment, they may meet some but not of the diagnostic criteria, they may have failed on other treatment regimens, and on and on. So an effectiveness study takes in anyone who, in actual practice, would be tried with that treatment.

In an efficacy trial, it makes sense to count only those people who have received the treatment as it should be given. That means that we would exclude, from the treatment group, those who died or dropped out, were lost to follow-up, didn't adhere to the treatment, and so forth. From the comparison group, we would exclude drop-outs, as well as those who, for one reason or another, received the active treatment.

On the other hand, in an effectiveness trial, we would use an **intention-to-treat (ITT)** approach—all people assigned to one arm would be counted in that arm, irrespective of what later happens to them. If a participant didn't fully comply, or if someone in the control group got the active treatment, or if people dropped out or died before the treatment kicked in, well, that's the way the of the world, and what would be expected when the intervention is used in the general population. The crunch comes at analysis time: How do we handle the missing data from those who dropped out or died? If the outcome is dichotomous, the most conservative approach is to say that everyone in the treatment group who dropped out got worse, and those in the comparison group got better. Dealing with continuous outcomes is far more problematic, and beyond the scope of this book. If you're really interested, take a look at *Biostatistics: The Bare Essentials* (Norman & Streiner, 2007).

SAMPLING

Needless to say, the most accurate information about the incidence of brain tumors in cell phone users would be gained if we could gather data from all cell phone users. Just as obviously, however, this would be impractical; there are millions of such users over most of the globe. Practical considerations dictate that we could follow up only a small proportion of these women, and if we select them appropriately, our estimates won't be off too far. (However, the famous prediction in 1936 that Alf Landon would decisively beat Franklin Roosevelt must serve as a constant reminder that "appropriately" isn't all that easy to define—much to Roosevelt's relief.) In this section, we discuss various ways in which we could go about choosing the group or groups we will include in our study.

Basic Terminology

Population
All of the people to whom the results should be applicable constitute the populations. In this example, the population would consist of all people who were regular users of cell phones (Figure 3-3). (Note that "population" does not refer to all the people in the world, just to those who have a specific disorder, were exposed to some agent, or underwent some procedure.)

Sample

In most cases the population is large, and it is impractical to study all people. We limit our study to a subset of the population; this smaller group is called the sample (Figure 3-4).

Cohort

You wouldn't want to meet a cohort in the original sense of the term; it was one-tenth of a Roman legion, composed of anywhere between 300 to 600 men, intent on pacifying the world through bloodshed, raping, and destruction—not exactly the image that epidemiology has of itself. What the cohort did have that was laudable was cohesion, and that's how we use the term today. When first introduced into the scientific lexicon, a cohort referred to a group of people born in the same time period; what we would now call a "birth cohort." Nowadays it has the broader, if less precise, meaning of a group of people who share some attribute. For instance, all people who began working at a specific job within a given time period can be referred to as a cohort, as can all people who entered the study at a certain time.

Probability Sampling

Probability sampling refers to a number of different strategies used to choose a sample. The term comes from the procedure used; every person in the population has a fixed and known probability of being selected to be

Figure 3-3. Example of a population.

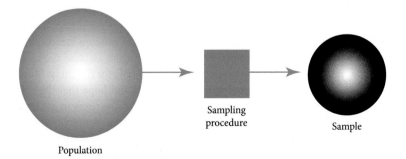

Figure 3-4. The sample is a subset of the population.

part of the sample. For a number of reasons, most studies try to use one or more of these strategies if at all possible.

The primary reason is that this method allows the investigator to generalize the results from the sample to the population, which is usually the major reason for doing a study. Second, it can tell the researcher the margin of error that could be expected from these estimates, that is, how far off the estimates can be. We see this in the reporting of polls, which often have a line stating that the results are accurate to within plus or minus 4%. In a related vein, most statistical tests are based on the assumption of some sort of random sampling. When probability sampling is not used, we shouldn't use these tests (although that has never stopped people from doing so), and the ability to generalize the results from the sample to the population is questionable. (This is in contrast to the view of one politician who trusted letters he received more than polls and complained that the latter were "only" random.)

Random Sampling

In **random sampling** (sometimes called "strictly random sampling" to differentiate it from the other varieties), each subject in the population has an equal chance of being chosen for the study. As we've mentioned, this approach maximizes the likelihood that the results of the study can be generalized to the entire population.

Random sampling is most often used in survey research (Figure 3-5). Nearly all towns and cities have lists of taxpayers (for obvious reasons) or of street and house addresses. This makes it relatively simple for the researcher to select people, or at least dwellings, at random. These days, approximately 98% of people have telephones, so it may seem as if it's easy to get a random sample from telephone lists or dialing numbers at random. But, more and more people are now relying solely on cell phones, making life more difficult, because the area codes and telephone numbers are not allocated on the basis of location. Further, people are being inundated with unsolicited calls during dinner or while they're watching their favorite TV show, making them less likely to respond to yet another unwanted solicitation from an interviewer.

Once we move out of the realm of surveys of the general population, however, it often becomes impossible to draw a pure random sample. We would have to know, for example, every person who had and had not used cell phones on a regular basis to select people randomly for the study. More often we choose one or a number of nearby cities and hope that the cell phone users within them are representative of cell phone users in general. We would then randomly select people within those cities for our sample.

The same situation exists even for experimentally based studies. The hospital where a new treatment is tried out is not really chosen at random; it is most likely selected on the basis of convenience (e.g., the investigator

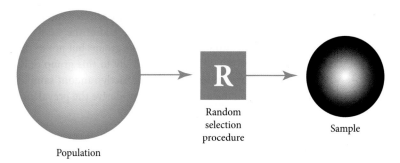

Figure 3-5. Random sampling.

works there or knows someone there who owes him or her a favor). The assumption is made that it is representative of hospitals in general and that the randomly selected patients from that hospital are representative of the general population of patients with that condition. Unfortunately, these assumptions are not always correct and result in many of the various types of selection biases, which we discuss starting on p. 63 in *Threats to Validity.*

Stratified Random Sampling

There are some circumstances in which we may wish to deviate from strictly random sampling. One major reason is that with random sampling, we may end up with too few people in one subgroup or another. For instance, if we thought that the effect of the phone was related to the placement of the antenna, random sampling might result in few left-handed people who have phones with extendable antennae; the sample would be too small to allow us to analyze the effects of antenna placement, free from the confounding influence that tumors may simply be more prevalent on one side of the brain. Similarly, we may want to have equal numbers of people who use regular as opposed to hand-free phones to maximize the power of our statistical tests.

Conversely, we may want to ensure that our sample is equivalent to the general population in terms of a few key variables, such as age at first using a cell phone or number of hours per week on the phone (although with teenagers, everyone may report 168 hours, which is the number of hours in a week). Random sampling ensures this matching in the long run with large enough samples, but not necessarily in our particular study, especially if there are fewer than 1000. By chance, we could over- or under-sample from a particular age or usage group.

To achieve these goals, we divide the key variables into various levels, or **strata**. For instance, we can divide age into 10-year increments or use into low, medium, and heavy (Figure 3-6). Then subjects are selected randomly from the stratum into which they fall. If toward the end of the study, we have enough people in the medium and heavy usage groups but not in the low use group, we would restrict entry into the study to this group only. Because we know how our strata deviate from a strictly random sample, we can correct for this during the analysis when we derive the prevalence figures.

Cluster Sampling

In some designs, it is impractical to assign individual subjects to the various groups. For example, in the Burlington Randomized Trial, nurse practitioners were placed in the offices of some family physicians to see whether they could reduce the cost of primary care without adversely affecting its quality. Outcome was measured at the level of the individual patient. However, because most families tend to use the same family physician, it would have been infeasible to allocate random members of the same family to different practices. In this case, each family was considered to be a **cluster**, and the unit of randomization was the family rather than the individual (Figure 3-7).

However, the two, three, or more people in the same household cannot be considered to be independent of one another in terms of health status; they share the same diet, environment, and likely have similar attitudes toward exercise or other behaviors that affect health. Consequently the husband's health is probably more correlated with his wife's than it is with that of another randomly chosen person.

Because the outcomes are correlated to some degree across people (who are usually considered to be independent in the usual statistical tests), studies that use cluster sampling usually need larger sample sizes than investigations in which the subjects are truly independent. How much larger the

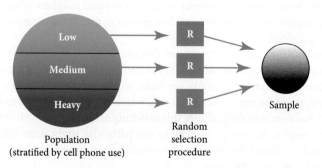

Figure 3-6. Stratified random sampling.

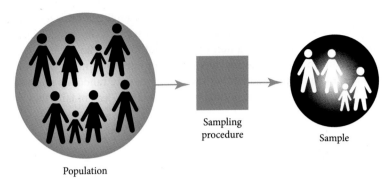

Population

Sampling procedure

Sample

Figure 3-7. Cluster sampling.

sample size has to be depends on the average number of people in the cluster and on how strongly the variables are correlated within members of the cluster.

Haphazard Sampling

In a **haphazard sample**, which is also called a "sample of convenience," subjects are selected on the basis of their availability or in any other non-random way. For example, a researcher can interview people who pass a certain street corner or take blood samples from the research assistants who work in his or her laboratory. There is always the real danger that this is a biased, nonrepresentative sample. During the day, housewives, shift workers, or the unemployed are more likely to be walking around outside than are people who work 9 to 5, and the location of the specific corner may differentially favor people from one social class over another. (On Wall Street in New York and Bay Street in Toronto, you were more likely to find yuppies in 1989 and the unemployed in 2009.) Similarly, those working in a laboratory may be healthier, brighter, or disproportionately female compared with the population of interest.

Unfortunately, newscasters rely on just this sort of haphazard "person in the street" interview to find out (often erroneously) what the people "really" think about some issue. Politicians who rely on letters they receive fall prey to the same trap; those who are concerned enough to write are not representative of the electorate in general. Lest we as researchers develop undue pride about our avoidance of such egregious errors as are committed by those who are untrained in the strict disciplines of science, two examples may suffice to remind us of our fallibility. Mueller and his colleagues developed a test for plasma unesterified fatty acid to be used for patients with neoplastic disease. Their 30 normal subjects were "members of the professional staff . . . or hospitalized normal volunteers." The sampling for this test may have been a marked improvement over another test, which studied hemolysate prothrombin consumption time; the authors gave no indication at all regarding how many normal blood samples were used, much less from where they came. To assume that these samples were randomly selected, and hence representative of normal people, requires a leap of faith that we at least cannot make.

SUBJECT ALLOCATION

As we have noted, in experimental studies, the researcher controls whether the person receives a treatment or some other intervention. Just as subjects can be *selected* for the study in various ways, they can be assigned or **allocated** to the different groups in a number of ways.

Sometimes these two steps are combined; as subjects are selected from the population, they are assigned to groups. In other instances, the two steps are explicitly differentiated; a sample is derived, and then a separate procedure is used to allocate the subjects to the various groups. However, it is important to be aware of these two steps, because many times, the first step (subject selection) is only implicit in the study. For example, although patients in a hospital can be randomly allocated to receive conventional therapy or a new treatment, there is actually an initial stage that may not have been acknowledged—namely, the selection of the hospitals where the study was carried out. In many instances, this initial selection procedure was not random.

Unfortunately, the similarity of terms used to describe subject selection and allocation can lead to considerable confusion for the uninitiated or unwary reader and offers an area of potential mischief for unscrupulous researchers (a group that fortunately does not include epidemiologists—often). In the previous example, the sample was randomly assigned to the treatment groups, but it was selected haphazardly. Describing the procedure as randomized, without adequately delineating the somewhat suspect origins of the sample, can be misleading.

Randomized Allocation

With random allocation, all subjects in the sample have the same probability of being assigned to the experimental group or to the control group. (This is not the same as a specific subject having an equal probability of being assigned to the groups; for design reasons, one group may be deliberately larger than the other, so the probability of ending up in that group is higher. However, the probability would be the same for all subjects.) This ensures that in the long run (i.e., with a large number of subjects), any underlying factors that may affect the outcome are equivalent for each group. There are two other advantages of this form of allocation. The first is that many of the statistical tests we use are based on the assumption of random assignment; violate this, and we can't trust the results of the tests. Second, it is the best way of preserving **blinding**, which means keeping people unaware of who gets what intervention (we'll discuss this in more detail a bit later).

Bear in mind that random selection and random allocation have different aims. As stated earlier, random *selection* of subjects is used to ensure the **generalizability** of the results from the sample to the population. The purpose of random *allocation* is to ensure the validity of any **cause-effect** interpretations we make from the data.

The subjects are allocated to groups by a **randomization device** or **scheme**. If there are only two groups that are equal in size, this can be accomplished by a simple coin toss: heads, then the first group; tails, the other group. However, it is more common to use a table of random numbers, which can be found in most introductory statistics books. These tables consist of many numbers, often listed in groups of 5 for the sake of readability, which are generated in a completely random fashion. An example of a small portion of a table of random numbers would look something like this:

92778	07201	92632	93521	18235
83855	98335	11980	90040	22843
85527	62908	55960	80310	46765
34606	20883	66096	23610	00765
37375	68228	49966	20361	57424
81839	59252	91022	94233	93928
67018	85005	03174	89887	94262

To assign subjects to two groups, the table is entered at random; if the first number is odd, for example, the subject is allocated to Group A, and if it is even, to Group B. The second subject is assigned in the same way on the basis of the next number in the table; "next" can mean moving your finger right, left, up, or down. When there are three groups, the subject is assigned to the first group if the number is 1, 2, or 3; to the second group if the number is 4, 5, or 6; and to the last group if the number is 7, 8, or 9. If a zero is encountered, it is simply ignored, and the next nonzero number is used. Groups of unequal sizes can be created in the same way. If Group A is to be twice the size of B, then numbers 1 through 6 can be used to allot subjects to Group A and 7 to 9 to Group B.

Now that you've mastered the arcane art of using tables of random numbers, the good news is that you probably won't need to do it, because most computers can easily produce random numbers. There are a number of programs that capitalize on this and produce lists of random assignments according to your specifications—equal numbers in all groups, one group twice the size of the others, and so on. However, they're based on the same principles as those of the random number table, so your mental effort was not in vain.

Bear in mind that what some people think is random allocation is really non-random. If people are assigned to groups on the basis of the day of the week they appear, then it's very easy to "game the system;" that is, to figure out into which group they'll end up. So, a referring physician, who wants to be sure that her patient gets the new, super-duper (but unproven) treatment will hold off referring the patient until it's the "right" day. Using the first letter of the patient's last name isn't much better—there'll be a preponderance of Scots and Irish in the group for M and O (not too many Dutch people have names starting with Mc or Mac or O'); and a disproportionate number of Jews with Rs (Rosenberg, Rosenbaum, Rosenzweig, and all their cousins).

Block Randomization

Block randomization is a modification of random allocation in which subjects are allocated in small blocks that usually consist of 2 to 4 times the number of groups (Figure 3-8). If there are three groups, then the block size is often 6, 9, or 12 subjects.

The subjects in the first block are randomly assigned so that there are equal numbers in each group (or, if the groups are not to be equal, they are assigned in proportion to the size of each group). The subjects in the succeeding blocks are then randomized in turn until the final sample size is achieved. (Figure 3-9).

Block randomization ensures that even if the study ends prematurely, there will be nearly equal numbers in all groups. If the sample size is small, it is possible to have a "run" of participants assigned to one group. For example, if the total sample size is 20, then there's about a 10% chance that you can end up with 3 or fewer people in one group and 7 or more in the other. This imbalance lowers the power of statistical tests, meaning that they're less likely to be significant when there actually is a difference between the groups. If you have sample sizes over 200 or so, this isn't an issue.

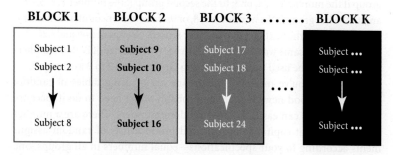

Figure 3-8. Allocation of subjects into blocks.

Figure 3-9. Block randomization.

Stratified Allocation

The aim of **stratified allocation** is slightly different from that of stratified selection. In the selection phase, stratification is used to ensure that the sample has certain desired characteristics. These characteristics may demand that the sample (1) matches the population on certain key variables, (2) includes sufficient numbers of subjects in all strata to permit subanalyses, or (3) has a normal distribution. The purpose of stratified allocations is more simple; it ensures that the groups do not differ too significantly on the stratification variables.

Stratified allocation is done when it is believed that the stratification variables may affect the outcome. If the groups are not balanced, any difference in outcome may result from these "nuisance" variables rather than from our intervention. For instance, if response to treatment is related to the patient's age, we do *not* want the experimental and control groups to differ on this factor.

For logistic reasons, it is often impractical to have more than two or three stratifying variables, unless the available population is large in relation to the sample size. Variables for stratification are chosen on the basis of their potential to affect the outcome. For example, because we felt that response to treatment was related to age but not to sex, only the former variable should be considered as a stratifying variable. If both age and duration of illness affect the outcome, but only one can be used as a stratification variable because of sample size limitations, the one that is more strongly associated with the outcome would be the variable to choose.

Bear in mind, though, that when the sample size is small, it may be hard to get the last few subjects to fill certain strata—that left-handed, 45-year-old, brown-eyed mother of three (adorable) kids. The good news is that while stratification is useful with small studies (fewer than about 50 people in each group), it is rarely worth the effort in larger trials; randomization usually is sufficient to balance the groups in terms of prognostic factors.

Minimization

Minimization is a very handy substitute for stratified randomization, especially when there are a number of variables that must be balanced between (or among) the groups, and the sample size is small. It gets its name from the allocation scheme, which tries to minimize differences between the groups on baseline characteristics. It's regarded as the one of the few legitimate non-random way of assigning people to groups. Let's say, in a hypothetical study, we have two groups of women—a treatment group and a control—and we want to make them as equivalent as possible in terms of parity, socioeconomic status (SES), and current smoking. Although statisticians tell us that we should never change a continuous variable into a categorical one, we'll ignore this advice (which we ourselves have given on countless occasions) and do just this, because for minimization, it makes our lives immeasurably easier. To keep it simple, we'll break parity into just two categories—0 previous kids, and one or more—and treat smoking as simply Yes or No. SES is a categorical variable to begin with, so we don't have to worry about it.

For the first few subjects, we'll just assign them to the two groups at random. Let's assume that after the first 10 participants, the situation looks like Table 3-1. Now the 11th person comes along, who has two kids at home, is in the middle class, and smokes. What we'll do is add up the number of people in each group with her characteristics. In the Treatment group, this would be:

$$3 \text{ (Parity} > 0) + 3 \text{ (Middle SES)} + 3 \text{ (Smoker)} = 9$$

and for the Control group:

$$2 \text{ (Parity} > 0) + 2 \text{ (Middle SES)} + 1 \text{ (Smoker)} = 5$$

so she would be assigned to the group with the smaller number in order to minimize the overall difference between the groups. If the numbers are equal, flip a coin. Now we update the table, and use the new numbers for the next person to come along.

Although the technique has been around for about 30 years, and researchers such as Taves have used it for balancing groups on the basis of 15 variables simultaneously, it isn't used too often. Part of the problem, at

Table 3-1
Characteristics of Two Groups After the First 10 Subjects

Variable	Treatment	Control
0 Kids	2	3
SES		
Low	1	2
Middle	3	2
High	1	1
Smoking - Yes	3	1

least until recently, may be the lack of programs to do the dirty work, but now many are freely available on the Web. Some people have also questioned whether statistics based on randomization can be used with minimization and, as far as we know, this is still up in the air.

Matching

The term **matching** can have two meanings: one applies at the level of the individual subject and the other describes the general strategy for selecting a control group.

Matching at the individual level means that a pair of experimental and control subjects are chosen to be as similar as possible in terms of certain key variables, such as age, sex, race, socioeconomic status, number of hospital admissions, or diagnosis. A person from the smaller subject pool is often chosen first (e.g., if there are fewer "exposed" than "nonexposed" people in a case-control design, the pool of potential experimental subjects is smaller than that of the controls). Then a subject from the other pool is selected and matched as closely as possible on the key characteristics. The larger the ratio of potential subjects to the desired number to be chosen, the more matching variables can be used. If there are not too many people to choose from, the number of matching variables must be reduced or the criteria for similarity are relaxed (e.g., matching for age within plus or minus 10 years rather than within 5). The result of matching is two groups that are as similar as possible on these key variables.

At the level of the group, matching refers to selecting a control group that has certain characteristics as an aggregate. For example, subjects in this control group can be (1) patients at the same hospital but with a different diagnosis, (2) drawn from the same community, or (3) working at similar jobs. Control subjects, however, are not matched to experimental subjects on a one-to-one basis.

The purpose of matching on certain variables is to eliminate the effect of those variables on group differences. If the two groups are matched on age, for example, any difference in outcome between the groups cannot result from this factor. The downside is that matching prevents us from examining at some later point the effect of age on the outcome. The moral is to match only when you're certain that you aren't ruling out examination of an association in which you may later be interested.

Groups are **undermatched** if they differ on some variable that is related to the outcome. The effect of undermatching is that group differences at the end may be caused by the variables that aren't matched. So there is a fine line between overmatching and thus being unable to explore potentially interesting relationships, and undermatching, which may cause your results to be explained by some extraneous variable.

Nonrandom (Haphazard) Allocation

Nonrandom allocation refers to situations in which participants end up in the various groups in some manner other than having been randomly assigned. Let's assume that we want to explore the hypothesis that exposure to fumes from copying machines has adverse consequences for pregnant women and their fetus. So, we could select workers at random from a bunch of offices in our city (stratified or otherwise), and then identify those who did copying and those who did not. We would then compare the Apgar scores of kids whose mothers did copying with a group of kids whose mothers didn't copy. Although we could *select* mothers at random from offices, the *allocation* would not have been random; the mothers would have been assigned to the copier based on their job description.

The difficulty here is that there may be other factors on which these two groups of people differ. Some factors to be taken into consideration include the following:

1. Working women may be healthier than women in general (see the discussion on subject selection biases in *Threats to Validity*).
2. They may be working because they are poorer than other women (or become richer because they are working) and therefore provide a different prenatal environment.
3. Even if we match for working status, those who are relegated to photocopying may differ in other regards from women who are managers or do the cleaning.

In brief, the investigator has no control over factors that may, on the one hand, determine group membership and, on the other hand, affect the outcome.

The problem is even more acute in therapy trials. Clinical factors, which are also related to outcome, may have dictated whether the patient received medical or surgical treatment for his or her condition or was given one drug rather than another. So simply comparing the success rates of these haphazardly selected groups may lead to erroneous results, because we conclude that the difference between the groups was caused by the intervention rather than by the factors that originally placed the subject in one group rather than in the other.

OTHER FORMS OF RANDOMIZATION

Despite the popularity of random allocation, there are a number of problems with it. First, if the new treatment is less effective than the traditional one, half of the subjects would be receiving less than optimum therapy. Conversely, if a new intervention is more effective than placebo, then the latter group has missed out on a chance to benefit. Second, because not all subjects who are approached agree to participate in a study and we know that volunteers are different from refusers (you'll know that, too, in another few pages), a high refusal rate can jeopardize the external validity of a trial (i.e., the extent to which the results can be generalized to the world at large). Through the years, a number of variations of randomization have been developed to try to overcome these shortcomings.

One group of procedures is referred to as **adaptive sampling**. This means simply that the allocation is adapted to match the results from people previously enrolled in the study. The best known procedure is **play the winner**, which is useful if (1) the outcome is a binary one, and (2) the results are known fairly quickly. We start off by assigning the first patient to either Treatment A or Treatment B at random; let's assume it was to Treatment B. If the outcome were positive, then the next patient would also be assigned to B, whereas if it were negative, the next patient would be enrolled in A. In this way, the more successful treatment will end up with the larger number of patients. In fact the difference in the proportion of patients allocated to each group is directly related to the magnitude of the treatment difference. The effect of this procedure then is to minimize the number of subjects receiving the less effective or more harmful treatment.

One problem with play the winner is that, after the first pair has been randomized, everyone else could end up in one group. In fact, that's exactly what happened in the ECMO trial: 11 neonates received extracorporeal membrane oxygenation and only one got the conventional treatment. Even putting aside the reservations of a trial with a total sample size of 12, not too many people were convinced by the results. So, a modification of play the winner is the **randomized play the winner**. Imagine an urn filled with an equal number (n) of balls that have either an A or a B on them, which indicates group membership. If the patient was successful on treatment A or failed with treatment B, then k balls marked A are added to the urn. Similarly, if the person did well on B or badly on A, then k B balls are thrown in. In this way, there is still a possibility that the next person on the list will get the poorer treatment, but the probability isn't zero, as it is with the unmodified play the winner method. The ratio of n to k affects how much the probability will be skewed toward the better treatment: as n is increased, it's closer to 50%; as k is increased, it shifts to favor the more successful treatment.

Another variant to random assignment is called **Zelen randomization**, which can be used when a new therapy is being tested against usual practice. Figure 3-10, *A*, shows what happens with the usual procedure: prospective patients are approached for their consent to be in a trial, and only those who agree are randomized to the treatment conditions. But why should people who end up receiving the usual form of care be approached for consent? If they refuse to participate in the study, they will be getting this anyway; all consent does is perhaps make them concerned about being in a study and makes a larger group of people eligible to refuse. Instead, Zelen randomization follows the procedure shown in Figure 3-10, *B*. Patients are first randomized, and only those allocated to the new treatment are approached for consent. This cuts down the number of people who can say "No."

This technique can work only if the control condition is usual practice and not placebo. Even so, there are some ethical problems in that the patients in the control group are in a study but haven't been told this. For this reason, there have been many articles written about Zelen randomization but few studies that have actually used it.

There are some other designs that overcome the limitations of Zelen randomization, and at the same time, take the patients' preferences into account while trying to increase the number of people who agree to participate. One is the **Zelen design with double randomization**, which is shown in Figure 3-11, *A*. First, patients are randomized to each condition and only

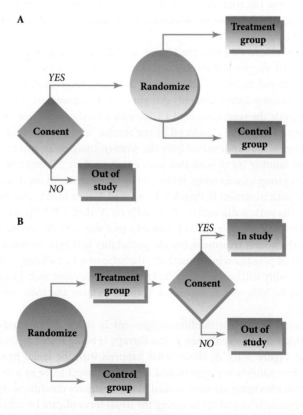

Figure 3-10. A, Regular and **B,** Zelen randomization.

afterward is consent sought. If they are happy with their assigned group, they remain in it; otherwise, they are switched to the other group. Because the patients know whether they're getting the new treatment or the standard one (or a placebo), blinding is compromised (we'll discuss the problems with that a bit later in the chapter). Consequently, this design works best in situations where blinding isn't possible, such as when the two treatment arms are a surgical versus a medical intervention, or group versus individual psychotherapy.

A **comprehensive cohort design** (Figure 3-11, *B*) combines elements of a randomized controlled trial (RCT) with a cohort study (terms that will be defined more a little later in the chapter). Patients are first asked if they'd be willing to be randomized to get either the new treatment or the comparator, just as in a usual RCT. In the traditional RCT, those who refuse randomization would simply be dropped from the study, leading to potential problems in terms of sample size, non-representativeness of people in the study, and so on. With this design, though, the refusers are assigned to the group of their choice, but analyzed separately. In this way, it's possible to see if those who agree to randomization differ from those who don't in terms of their outcome.

Finally, in the **Wennberg design** (Figure 3-11, *C*), patient preferences are dealt with more explicitly. They are first asked if they would be willing to

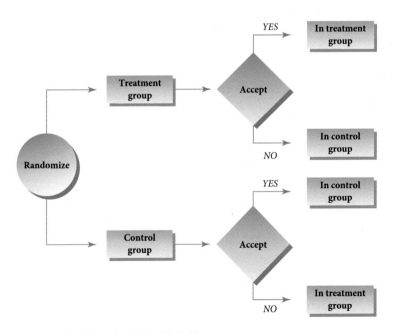

Figure 3-11A. Zelen randomization with double consent.

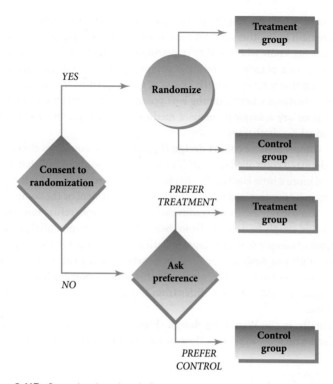

Figure 3-11B. Comprehensive cohort design.

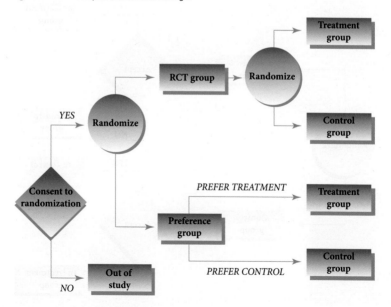

Figure 3-11C. Wennberg's design.

be randomized into either (a) an RCT, or (b) a condition in which they can choose the intervention. If they agree, then the RCT people are randomized yet again to receive the treatment or the comparator; while those in the preference group make their own choice. As with the comprehensive cohort design, the groups are analyzed separately to see if the patient characteristics that influenced the initial choice affected the outcome. It is likely that as patients demand more of a role in determining what happens to them, this design will become more popular.

THREATS TO VALIDITY

The purpose of any study is to tell us what is "really" happening in the world: Does streptokinase reduce cardiac mortality? What causes sudden infant death syndrome? Did the swine flu vaccination program do more good than harm? We hope that the results from our sample can be generalized to the population at large so that our findings also hold true for similar people. Consequently it is disconcerting, at the least, to find different studies coming to opposite conclusions.

The major reason for these differences is that all studies have flaws involving (1) the definition of the disorder or phenomenon of interest, (2) the selection of the subjects, or (3) the design or execution of the study itself. Cook and Campbell call these flaws **threats to validity**. In this discussion, we examine some of the more common ones and see how they can affect the interpretation of the results. In Chapter 4, we discuss those forms of bias that affect eliciting and recording information.

Internal and External Validity

Cook and Campbell make a very useful distinction between two classes of threats to the validity of a study—**internal validity** and **external validity**. Before discussing these, though, we should point out that the term "validity" is most often used in the context of developing outcome measures (a topic we'll discuss in Chapter 4). It has a related meaning when it's used to discuss the design of studies—how much we can trust that the findings are true and apply in our settings—but the technical details are quite different. However, stay tuned and all will be made perfectly clear.

Internal validity is concerned with the design of the study, and how various biases can jeopardize the conclusions. Many studies try to answer one or both of two questions: (a) are two variables related to each other; and (b) if so, is the relationship a causal one? A lack of internal validity can give us the wrong answer to both questions, and in both directions—masking relationships that actually exist, and producing relationships when in fact there aren't any. There are, sadly, many threats to internal validity, and this is only a partial listing.

Statistical Threats

A full discussion of this belongs in a statistics book (that's is a plug to read *PDQ Statistics*), but it's useful to know what types of threats exist. These include (a) too few subjects to show a significant effect (what is called *power*); (b) violating the assumptions of statistical tests; (c) going on a fishing expedition by blindly testing everything that moves; and (d) using unreliable outcome measures, which we'll discuss in Chapter 4.

Treatment Implementation

Not standardizing how the intervention is give from one participant to the next.

History and Maturation

These are a problem in longitudinal studies, when people are studied over time. Something may change between assessment times, either externally (history) or within the person (maturation) that can account for difference (e.g., change in diagnostic practices or treatment; participants becoming familiar with the scales; or just getting older).

Selection

A particular problems in case-control and cohort studies, and other quasi-experimental designs, whereby the people in one group differ in some systematic ways from those in the other group.

Drop-Outs

If people drop out of a study, then those who remain may be different from those who drop out. This is magnified if people drop out of various groups for different reasons and at different rates.

Diffusion or Imitation of Treatment

If people in an experimental condition talk to those in the control group, then the latter may adopt some aspects of the intervention. For example, if a new program is implemented with nurses on one unit in a hospital, they may talk over lunch to nurses from other units, who then begin to introduce the new procedures.

Compensatory Equalization of Treatments

Wittingly or unwittingly, those in the comparison group get other interventions to compensate for the fact that they're not getting the new treatment. For instance, if one group gets an add-on medication and starts to improve, the staff may give other treatments to those in the comparison group.

External validity asks about the generalizability of the findings from the study to the population at large, across different people, settings, and times. The major threat to external validity is non-random sampling. We have already discussed some aspects of this, and the next section will go into more detail about other aspects of it, so there's no need to elaborate here. What should be emphasized, though, is that there is often a reciprocal relationship between internal and external validity—as we improve one, we often decrease the other. For example, one excellent way to increase the internal validity of experiments and medical trials is to make the groups as homogeneous as possible. This reduces the variability within the groups, making it more likely to find statistical significance, and hence reducing the statistical threats to validity. Needless to say, though, this then limits the generalizability of the findings to other people. Similarly, we can maximize treatment implementation validity by using only the most experienced clinicians; giving them extra training and supervision in the technique we're investigating; and so on. Again, though, the cost is a reduction in external validity because, Lake Wobegon notwithstanding, not every clinician is above average. The art in designing studies is finding the balance between external and internal validity.

Subject Selection Biases

Subject selection biases involve a host of factors that may result in the subjects in the sample being unrepresentative of the population. We've already discussed one class of selection bias—non-random sampling. However, even with the best of sampling strategies, nature (human and otherwise) conspires against us in many ways. Sackett compiled a list of various biases, 57 at last count, and even this is probably incomplete. To keep life simple, we can think of two major types of subject selection biases: who gets *invited* to participate in a study and who *accepts*. We cannot even attempt to provide a complete catalog of these two classes of factors; rather, the following three examples of invitational bias (healthy worker, incidence-prevalence, and Berkson's) and one of acceptance bias (volunteer) are illustrative only. We hope these examples help enlighten and warn the reader of where things can go wrong.

Healthy Workers Bias

Random sampling does not help us if the group from which the sample is drawn is unrepresentative of the population to which we want to generalize. For example, comparing the outcome of pregnancies of women who work with copying machines with those of a group of women chosen at random may open up the researcher to the **healthy worker bias**; that is, people who work are, as a group, healthier than the population as a whole. The entire adult population consists of those people who are working, those who are able to work but do not for one reason or another, and those who cannot work because of health problems. Any group of workers, by definition, does not include this last category of people that tends to lower the overall health status of the population. This selection bias operates even more strongly when the job applicants have to pass a physical examination, as in the Armed Forces or certain labor-intensive occupations. Seltzer and Jablon, for example, found lower morbidity rates among people discharged from the army than among people of similar ages in the general population. This effect was seen even 23 years after the men had been discharged. (Some have hypothesized that this is caused by army food killing off the less-fit before they can be discharged.)

The effects of this bias are to (1) make any sample drawn from a group of workers appear healthier than the general population; (2) make the standardized mortality rate (see Chapter 4) less than 1:1 when workers are compared with the general population; and (3) make the proportional mortality rate (see Chapter 4) for occupational hazards greater than 1.0 because of "borrowing" (i.e., if they are dying less from heart disease, they must be dying more from something else).

Incidence-Prevalence (Neyman) Bias

If a group is investigated a significant amount of time after the people have been exposed to a putative cause or after the disorder has developed, those who have died and those who have recovered will be missed. This is known as **incidence-prevalence** bias or the **Neyman** bias. For example, a cross-sectional look at depressed patients in hospital misses those in whom the depression culminated in suicide or resolved itself. Similarly, a study of cardiac patients in a tertiary care hospital does not include (1) those who died before reaching hospital and (2) those whose myocardial infarction was not sufficiently severe to warrant transfer to a specialized facility.

As another example, even the latest version of the *Diagnostic and Statistical Manual of Mental Disorders* (2000) is somewhat pessimistic regarding the long-term prognosis in schizophrenia. However, this pessimism may be unwarranted and may be based on the fact that most "natural history" studies use patients who are in hospital at a given time. Follow-up studies with patients who have been admitted for the first time, which are much less susceptible to the Neyman bias than cross-sectional ones, give a different picture; according to these follow-up studies, the majority of patients— anywhere between 60 and 80%—go on to lead productive lives outside the hospital.

The effects on the Neyman bias can be in two different directions. Missing those who died before they could be included in the study makes the disorder look less severe because the outcome is generally more positive than had all patients been included. Conversely, missing those who have already gotten better makes the outcome look grimmer. The net effect is often unknowable and depends on the relative proportions of patients in the three groups (i.e., studied, died, and improved).

Berkson's Bias

Berkson's bias is the spurious association found between some characteristic and a disease, and it results from admission rates to hospital (or any other setting where the study is carried out) being different for those persons (1) with the disease, (2) without the disease, and (3) with the characteristic. For example (Table 3-2), assume that in the general population there is no relationship at all between vaginal bleeding (the characteristic) and endometrial cancer (the disease).

Let us further assume that 10% of patients with endometrial cancer have vaginal bleeding and 10% of patients with other cancers have bleeding. If the probability of being admitted to hospital because of vaginal bleeding is 70%, if it's 10% because of endometrial cancer and if it's 50% because of other of cancer, then we we can assume the following:

1. Of the 100 patients with vaginal bleeding and endometrial cancer (cell A), 10 will be admitted because of endometrial cancer (i.e., 10%). Of the remaining 90 patients in cell A, 63 (70%) will be admitted because of vaginal bleeding, so that a total of 73 women will be admitted with endometrial cancer and bleeding.
2. Of the 100 patients with vaginal bleeding and other forms of cancer (cell B), 50 will be admitted because of the other cancers. Of the remaining

Table 3-2
Association Between Endometrial Cancer and Vaginal Bleeding

		Type of Cancer		
		Endometrial	Other	
Vaginal Bleeding	Yes	100 (A)	100 (B)	200
	No	900 (C)	900 (D)	1800
		1000	1000	2000

50, 35 (again, 70%) will be admitted because of vaginal bleeding, so that in total 85 will be admitted with bleeding and other cancers.

3. Of the 900 patients with endometrial cancer and no bleeding (cell C), 90 (again, 10%) will be admitted because of endometrial cancer.

4. Of the 900 patients with other forms of cancer and no bleeding (cell D), 450 will be admitted because of the other cancers.

Table 3-3 shows the graphic results of these different admission rates. Now it appears that 44.8% of patients with endometrial cancer have vaginal bleeding, whereas only 15.9% of patients with other forms of cancer have vaginal bleeding. This apparent (and false) association is the result of different hospitalization rates for endometrial and other cancers and for vaginal bleeding. Thus Berkson's bias comes into play whenever we sample from a setting in which there are different rates of admission for different disorders.

The bias also occurs within the same disorder, when patients with more symptoms are hospitalized at a higher rate than patients with fewer symptoms. For example, schizophrenics with both positive symptoms (e.g., hallucinations) and negative symptoms (apathy) are more likely to end up in hospital than those with only one of these sets of symptoms. The result is that the association between the two is much higher than in patients living in the community.

Volunteer Bias

To be ethical, most studies allow patients to refuse to participate. Thus the results are predicated to some degree on the assumption that those who do not volunteer are similar to those who do. However, there is now ample evidence to show that this is not the case and that volunteers differ systematically from nonvolunteers.

Table 3-3
Results Caused by Different Hospitalization Rates for Characteristic (Bleeding) and Disease (Cancer)

		Type of Cancer		
		Endometrial	Other	
Vaginal Bleeding	Yes	73 (A)	85 (B)	158
	No	90 (C)	450 (D)	540
		163	535	698

For example, the National Diet-Heart Study found that, compared with nonvolunteers, volunteers more frequently (1) were nonsmokers, (2) were concerned about health matters, (3) had a higher level of education, (4) were employed in professional and skilled jobs, (5) were Protestant or Jewish, (6) were living in households with children, and (7) were active in community affairs.

Not surprisingly, a similar problem exists when we're trying to track people down, either to find out what happened to them or to ask them some questions as part of a survey; those who are harder to find are different from people who can be contacted more easily. What may be surprising is that this is an issue even for those who have gone to meet the great epidemiologist in the sky. The mortality rate among neurotic patients who were easy to trace was 2.7%; for those who were more difficult to locate, it shot up to 27.3%.

An analogous sort of effect, which we could probably name **compliance bias**, exists among those who participate in trials. In one arm of the Coronary Drug Project, the 5-year mortality rate for compliers (those who took 80% or more of their medication) was 15.1%. It was almost twice as high among noncompliers (28.2%), even though the "medication" they were complying with was a placebo. Similarly the mortality rate in the β-Blocker Heart Attack Trial was twice as high for noncompliers, whether they were adhering to taking their propranolol or their placebo. Although all subjects were volunteers in both of these trials, those who complied with the treatment regimen were apparently a different breed from those who did not comply.

Even for those who participate in a trial, a type of volunteer bias may operate. The incidence of inactive tuberculosis was lower among volunteers who appeared early during a mass screening than among those who appeared later, whereas the opposite trend was noted for pneumoconiosis.

Biases Affecting the Outcome

Just as there are biases that affect who gets into a study, there are other biases that may distort the outcomes. Some of these, such as the Hawthorne Effect, influence how people behave during the study; while others, such as a lack of blinding, proxy measures, and recall bias, affect what is recorded. In either case, though, the internal validity of the study can be seriously compromised.

Hawthorne Effect

According to legend, worker productivity improved at the Hawthorne plant of the Western Electric Company not only when the illumination was increased but also later when it was decreased. The reason for this was supposed to be the attention paid to the workers by the researchers and not the lighting itself. Although later studies showed that the increase in productivity likely resulted from other factors, the term **Hawthorne effect** has remained to explain the phenomenon that occurs when a subject's performance changes simply because he or she is being studied (some have erroneously referred to this as the psychological equivalent of the Heisenberg Uncertainty Principle).

For example, Frank reported that the introduction of a research project onto a hospital ward was "followed by considerable behavioral improvement in the patients," even though no medication or special treatments were involved. He felt that the most likely explanation was that "participation in the project raised the general level of interest of the treatment staff, and the patients responded favorably to this."

To counteract the Hawthorne effect it is often necessary to use an *attention control group*, which is treated exactly the same as the experimental group except for the active treatment. For example, studies of psychotherapy often use a control group that meets with the therapist as frequently and for the same duration as does the treatment group, but the content of the session is not supposed to be therapeutic. In drug trials the control group receives a placebo, which usually involves taking the same number of pills at the same time of day as the experimental subjects.

Blinding

One effect of the attention control group we just discussed is to **blind** the subject and perhaps the experimenter. A person is considered blind if he or she is unaware of the group to which a subject belongs. If only the subject is unaware but the experimenter knows, the study is called single blind. If both the subject and the researcher do not know, the study is labeled **double blind**. (Some people have proposed the term "triple blind" for the occasions when the subject and evaluator are blind, and the pharmacist has lost the key that tells who got the drug and who got the placebo. However, this is more a threat to the pharmacist's life than to validity.)

The purpose of blinding is to prevent various biases from affecting the results. Subjects may show a *placebo effect* if they know they are receiving an active agent or may not show it if they think they are not receiving the new drug. With single blinding, both groups should show an equivalent reaction. The magnitude of the placebo effect should not be underestimated (indeed, it's what kept medicine alive for a few millennia). The results of one typical study, shown in Figure 3-12, indicate that more than 50% of patients experienced relief of headache pain from placebos.

If the clinicians (or evaluators) were aware of group membership, they could be more alert or attentive to signs of improvement. Likewise,

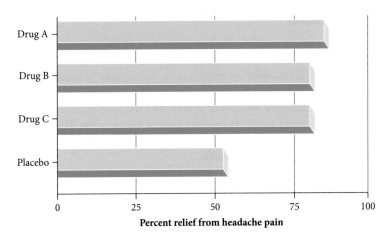

Figure 3-12. Results of this study show the placebo effect. In this case more than 50% of subjects on placebo experienced relief of headache pain. (From Beecher HK: The powerful placebo, JAMA 159:1602–1606, 1955.)

clinicians who know that a disease should be present may be more diligent when looking for it (*diagnostic suspicion bias*). Rosenthal conducted a series of studies that showed that what a researcher expects to find in an experiment affects what does occur, irrespective of whether the subjects are humans or rats.

Although blinding is a critical element of good experiments, there are times when it's hard to put into practice. Blinding works well when it's a matter of making up clever little pill bottles with little codes in the corner, but if one drug makes you tired, or makes your urine green, or makes your hair fall out, then all is for naught. And when we go beyond pills, it gets very difficult to ensure blinding. In surgery, the scar is a dead giveaway. There was one trial years ago where everyone got the surgery but in the control group the artery wasn't ligated, but that doesn't happen often today. In reality, just about every non-pharmacological intervention is hard to blind. Chiropractic? Well, it can be done occasionally: Balon compared sham chiropractic, which broke the historical rules of chiropractic, to the real thing, for treatment of asthma. Everyone in the chiropractic group got better; so did everyone in the sham group. But in general, it's hard to avoid having folks know what's going on.

One of us (Geoff Norman) does research in education, and is regularly berated for not doing more RCTs. While some experimentation is likely a good thing, it will be a weird day indeed when we manage to pull off an educational intervention where no one is aware they received it. Regrettably, it is not easy to determine the degree of unblinding in any study (unless it's 100%), and even harder to figure out how to correct for it.

Proxy Measures

Proxy measures are variables, both dependent and independent, that stand in for other variables. They're used for two reasons. The first, and more legitimate one, is that what we really want to look at may be too difficult to measure directly because it is too invasive to do so (e.g., density of neural plaques in Alzheimer's disease) or it may take too long to manifest itself (such as death), and so on. The second reason, which is less defensible, is that we're not aware that we're dealing with proxy measures. Let's start off by looking at the dependent variable.

Surrogate End Points

Imagine that you've discovered a new drug that promises to reduce cardiac mortality by raising the levels of "good" cholesterol among otherwise healthy women. However, you quickly find out that in order to see if the treatment, which you've called "LiDLe Women" works, you'll have to enroll 20,000 subjects and follow them for 30 years. Because the Tenure and Promotions Committee meets to decide your fate next year, you can't wait that long. Part of the problem, about which you can do nothing, is that the rate of cardiac deaths among young women is low. The other factor contributing to the large sample size requirement is that you're looking at a dichotomous outcome—alive or dead. As you'll see in the next chapter, you need far fewer subjects if you measure the outcome on a continuum so you look around for some end point that can be measured this way and come up with an index of coronary artery stenosis. Congratulations! You have just played the surrogate end point game.

Stenosis, diastolic blood pressure, or CD4+ cell counts among acquired immunodeficiency syndrome (AIDS) patients are surrogate measures because, when we come right down to it, changing the values of these measures isn't what the therapies really concern. We are interested in them only to the degree that they are correlated with the true outcome, which in these cases is death. If there is a strong association between the surrogate and the actual outcome of interest, then using a proxy can result in shorter trials with fewer patients and for far less money. However, if the relationship is weak, despite what our theory tells us, then we can come to wrong conclusions. For example, the Cardiac Arrhythmia Suppression Trial tried to reduce premature ventricular contractions (PVCs) because it was believed that suppressing them would result in fewer deaths. The good news is that the drugs did suppress PVCs; the bad news is that these patients died at a rate 2½ times that of the control group. And paralleling our fictitious example, a large study in Finland succeeded in reducing the risk factors for cardiovascular disease by 46% in the treatment group. Unfortunately, the men in that group died of heart disease at more than twice the rate as that in die control group. The problem with the arrhythmia trial was that they chose the wrong surrogate—it's atrial contractions that kill us, not ventricular ones. Nobody knows what the problem was in Finland. But a more subtle, and insidious, problem is when the surrogate works for one drug regimen but not another. To test the effects of the calcium channel blocker, nefidipine, researchers looked at blood pressure (a nice, continuous measure), rather than heart attacks (rare and dichotomous). That surrogate outcome measure worked fine at low doses of the drug—people had both lower blood pressure and a lower mortality rate—but people taking the highest doses of the drug died at a rate three times higher than the controls.

The moral of this tale is that surrogate end points can lead to more efficient trials, but they must have been proven to be closely associated with the true outcome. Reliance on theory or clinical supposition alone is never sufficient.

Surrogate Explanatory Variables

Often we see among the list of explanatory variables ones like sex, education, marital status, income, or ethnicity. These tend to be proxy measures of the second type, variables that we're not aware are actually stand-ins for other variables. But if we think about it a bit, we'll see that we are rarely interested in these variables in their own right. For example, many studies have documented the inverse relationship between income (or socioeconomic status) and health. But, as seen in countries with universal health insurance (e.g., Canada, Great Britain), money does not buy health. Rather, income is a measure of large differences in "lifestyle" factors between richer and poorer people that affect health, running the gamut from jobs (low-paying jobs tend to be more dangerous than office work), to nutrition, to smoking status. Similarly, when studies report differences in compliance rates between men and women, it is highly doubtful that they are postulating a biologic explanation of why women take medication more regularly than men. Here, gender is a proxy for other factors, such as socialization, relationships with authority figures, or concern about health.

The problems with using surrogate explanatory variables are at least twofold. First, we may be fooling ourselves about what the important factors are and how modifiable they are. We cannot change gender, for example, but we can alter attitudes toward health. Second, any time we measure a variable, we introduce measurement error. With proxy variables, we are introducing error upon error—the error of the measure and the degree to which the proxy is not a perfect indicator of the underlying variable that interests us.

Recall Bias

In many types of studies, we ask the participants to tell us what happened to them some time in the past, such as how often they saw their family doctor in the last year, whether they've ever been in hospital, what they ate during the past week, and so on. Needless to say, we expect that the answers will be both truthful and accurate. Poor deluded us! In Chapter 4, we'll discuss some of the factors, conscious and unconscious, that may distort the person's reporting; here, we'll focus on a seemingly simpler issue—how accurately people recall events. The answer is not encouraging; after reading this, you may decide to never ask anyone about anything.

Even when people mean to be honest and truthful (which isn't very often), recall is distorted by many factors. The first is simply the fallibility of memory. Difficult as it may be for us to imagine, a significant proportion of people in a large, population-based study forgot that they had been in hospital during the past year. Before you dismiss this as ridiculous, talk to anyone who has done a surgery rotation. How many times have they asked the patient, "Have you had any previous surgeries?" to which the patient says, "No, doc; this is the first one." Then in the OR, they whip off the surgical gown to find scars from a previous appendectomy, cholecystectomy, oophorectomy, and who knows what other ectomy. A second issue is that we ask people to remember events within the framework of a calendar—the last week, month, or year. But, memory isn't organized this way in our brain; it's arranged by salient events in our lives—"When I had this job," "When I was married to that person," "When I owned that real clunker of a car," or "When the kids still lived at home."

We also know that current events, especially illnesses, affects recall of past events. When something bad happens to us or our kids, we search back to find the ostensible reason. For example, mothers of children with congenital malformations reported using more drugs during pregnancy than did mothers of normal kids, although the log books kept during the pregnancy by the obstetricians showed no such difference.

Diagnostic Suspicion Bias

Under certain circumstances the rate of occurrence of a diagnosis can depart from expectations simply because of an enhanced index of suspicion on the part of the diagnostician. This bias may be highly individualized and short-term. One well-documented bias of individuals is illustrated by the clinical anecdote that goes something like this: "The funniest thing happened. Saturday night in the ER I diagnosed the first case of Somaliland camelbite fever I've seen in 20 years. This week I saw four more cases in my office. There must be a real epidemic going around!" A more likely explanation is the *availability bias*. The one case in the ER is readily available in memory and is likely to be recalled when anything similar comes along.

A more long-term and widespread diagnostic suspicion bias is the *syndrome syndrome*. Throughout the decades it is easy to show how the popularity of certain diseases has waxed and waned. In the 1920s a common syndrome was "self-pollution," or masturbation. The clinical syndrome was well described, and there were literally institutions filled with depraved little self-polluters. In fact, W. K. Kellogg ran a sanatorium for these lost souls in Battle Creek, Michigan and fed them Corn Flakes to suppress their carnal desires.

Lest you feel this is a perversion of the early days of medicine before the advent of sophisticated diagnostic procedures, there are many current examples. Alzheimer's disease has apparently reached epidemic proportions. Some of the increased incidence is a result of better diagnostic tools and more old people around to develop it. Nevertheless, the syndrome was first described in the early 1900s. Presumably, until recently, doddery old ladies were simply passed off as doddery old ladies. Now, if anyone over 65 forgets where they left their car keys, Alzheimer's is the first diagnosis to spring to mind.

We also alluded to the urea formaldehyde foam insulation (UFFI) issue earlier. The interesting tale about UFFI is that it was installed for several decades in Europe before its arrival in North America. Once here, relatively few problems arose until the media announced all the lethal consequences of the stuff. Following that point physicians everywhere were diagnosing any number of complaints, from headaches to ingrown toenails, as resulting from UFFI poisoning.

In the Preface, we mentioned one study in which physicians "found" tonsillitis requiring surgery in approximately 45% of kids, even when two other sets of physicians declared the kids clean (or at least not ill). Here again the expectation of finding a disorder biased what was seen by the physicians.

Confounding

Confounding is the illusory association between two variables when in fact no such association exists. It is caused by a third variable (the "confounder"), which is correlated with the first two. For example, Table 3-4 shows bifocal use (needed or not) and nocturnal enuresis (present or absent) in a group of 200 patients.

The odds ratio is 2.36, which indicates that persons who need bifocals are twice as likely to have enuresis as those who don't need bifocals. (This may be related to the supposed link between masturbation and blindness.)

However, a closer look at these data shows that there are actually two age groups involved (Table 3-5). For each age group, there is no association between bifocal use and enuresis. In those less than 60 years of age, 5% of bifocal users are enuretic (1 of 20 subjects), as are 5% of nonusers (4 of 80 subjects). For those more than age 60, 20% are enuretic, irrespective of bifocal use. The confounder here is age; bifocal users are more apt

Table 3-4

Relationship Between the Need for Bifocals and Nocturnal Enuresis

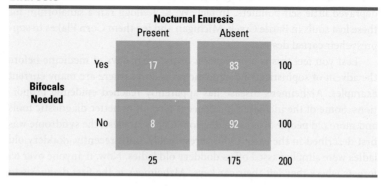

	Nocturnal Enuresis		
	Present	Absent	
Bifocals Needed Yes	17	83	100
No	8	92	100
	25	175	200

Table 3-5

No Association Between Bifocal Need and Nocturnal Enuresis When Subjects are Divided by Age

	Nocturnal Enuresis Less than Age 60			Nocturnal Enuresis More than Age 60		
	Present	Absent		Present	Absent	
Bifocals Needed Yes	1	19	20	16	64	80
No	4	76	80	4	16	20
	5	95	100	20	80	100

to be more than age 60, which is also the group that has the higher rate of enuresis (Figure 3-13).

To be a confounder, a variable must meet two criteria: (1) it must be a risk factor for the outcome of interest, and (2) it must be associated with the independent variable or distributed differently between the groups. Age meets these conditions, in that it is a risk factor for enuresis and is also related to the need for bifocals. We can control for confounders in a number of ways. If we were doing a study that allowed us to assign patients to groups, we could hope that **randomization** would balance the groups in terms of the confounder. If we cannot randomize or if we don't want to rely on it alone to ensure balanced groups, we can **match** on the variable; in this case, for each person who needs bifocals, we would choose a person to be in the nonbifocal group who is the same age, ensuring that the groups do not differ on this variable. Third, we can **stratify** on that variable by dividing the pool of subjects in each group into a number of age strata and sampling equal numbers per group from each stratum. If we were a bit lazier (or had a smaller pool of potential subjects from which to draw), we could **frequency match**. Here, we would ensure that the proportion of people of different ages were the same in the two groups, without being concerned that a specific person in one group was paired with someone in the other group. We would be satisfied if the overall proportions or frequencies were the same. However, matching raises some problems in the analysis stage and can be costly. Last, we could try to account for the differences between the groups **statistically**, by using the confounder as a *covariate* (a term that we explain in some detail in *PDQ Statistics* and *Biostatistics: The Bare Essentials*). Statisticians still argue vehemently among themselves whether any post hoc statistical manipulation can adequately control for preexisting differences between groups on some confounding variable. However, most of us blithely continue to do it, most likely because no potential subjects are lost because a similar person for the other group could not be found for them, as can easily happen with matching.

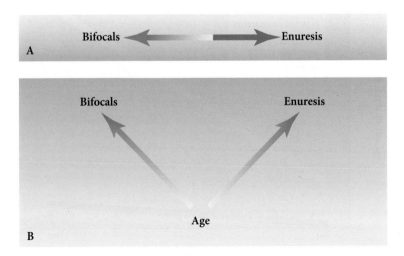

Figure 3-13. A, When unaware of the confounder, it appears that there is a direct association between enuresis and bifocals. **B**, There is a direct association between age (confounder) and bifocals and between age and enuresis.

Interactions

Often people use the term **confounding** when they really mean **interaction**. At one level, it's easy to see why—both are *effect modifiers*; that is, they modify the strength of the association between two variables. However, they're different animals. As we just saw, a confounder is a third variable that can produce an illusory association between two other variables or result in an apparent lack of association. An interaction, as the name implies, means that the effect of Variable A depends on the value of Variable B. For example, does oral contraceptive use increase the risk of heart attacks among women?

Figure 3-14, modified from Shapiro et al. (1979), shows the risk of myocardial infarctions (MIs) for women who use oral contraceptives and those who don't and for women who smoke to varying degrees, as compared with nonsmokers who are not taking oral contraceptives (i.e., their risk is 1.0). Does the risk increase? It all depends. If the women smoke fewer than 25 cigarettes a day (it's assumed they don't smoke cigars or pipes), then there is no appreciable increase in risk. However, if they smoke 25 cigarettes or more a day, their risk jumps from 7 times that of the nonsmokers (that's the effect of smoking) to 39 times. Therefore there is an interaction between oral contraceptive use and smoking in terms of the risk of MI: no increase for nonsmokers, and more than a five-fold risk for smokers. This means that one

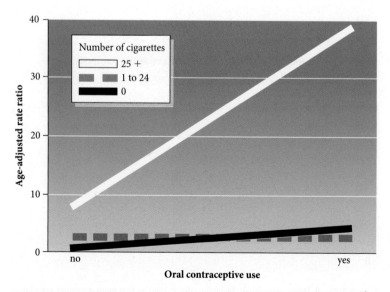

Figure 3-14. Interaction between oral contraceptive use and smoking in risk for heart attack. (Modified from Shapiro S, Slone D, Rosenberg L: Oral contraceptive use in relation to myocardial infarction, Lancet i:743–764, 1979.)

variable cannot be looked at in isolation; the overall risk is too high for those who smoke less than a pack a day and too low for those who smoke more.

Contamination

In studies in which one group receives the experimental treatment and another group gets either conventional treatment or a placebo, the validity of the results is predicated on the *purity* of the groups. If some subjects in the control group receive the new treatment, both groups will improve to some degree (assuming that the treatment works). Thus differences between the groups are diminished or even eliminated. This condition is referred to as **contamination** (what Cook and Campbell call "diffusion or imitation of treatment," which we mentioned earlier).

Contamination is a particular problem when a medication used in a study is also available over the counter or as an ingredient in other compounds (e.g., aspirin) or when it can be prescribed by family physicians who are unaware (or have forgotten) that certain drugs should not be given to some of their patients. However, contamination is not limited to drug trials; it can occur with any form of intervention, such as respite care for those taking care of demented elderly, psychotherapy, and similar maneuvers in which subjects in the control group receive some form of the treatment.

In cohort and case-control studies contamination is caused by misclassification, that is, assigning exposed subjects to the nonexposed group or vice versa. This is often caused by errors in recall by the subjects.

The effect of contamination is to reduce differences between the treated and untreated groups. This may lead us to draw the erroneous conclusion that the intervention is of limited or no use.

Cointervention

Cointervention ("compensatory equalization of treatments," in Cook and Campbell's jargon) refers to subjects in a study receiving therapies other than those given as part of the experiment that affect the outcome of interest. For example, some subjects in a study that compares the effectiveness of various nonsteroidal antiinflammatory drugs for arthritis could be given other drugs by another physician, be enrolled in a program using transcutaneous stimulation, or might be taking over-the-counter aspirin.

Cointervention differs from contamination in two ways: (1) the intervention and (2) the groups that are affected. First, contamination refers to the control group receiving the experimental intervention, whereas cointervention refers to some treatment other than the one under investigation. Second, all groups in a study can be witting or unwitting recipients of a certain cointervention, but only the control group can be contaminated.

Although all groups can be subject to cointervention, it is a particular danger when the control subjects do not improve or even deteriorate on placebo. If any other clinician is involved in the case and unaware of the study, he or she may prescribe other treatments to help the person, thereby minimizing differences between the groups. If subjects in all groups receive other therapies, then it becomes almost impossible to determine whether the results are caused by the treatment under study, by the cointervention, or by both.

Regression Toward the Mean

Regression toward the mean refers to the phenomenon whereby groups of subjects that are chosen because of their extreme score on any variable will have scores that are less extreme and closer to the mean value when they are retested. The reason is that any test result we observe—some serum value, a decision based on a radiograph, or a score on a paper and pencil test—is comprised of two parts: the *true* score and the *error* score. Written out in the form of an equation, we say the following:

$$\text{Observed Score} = \text{True Score} \pm \text{Error Component}$$

There are many sources of error (see Chapter 4), including variations in the machine, biologic variation within the subject, motivation, fatigue, and recording error. The assumption is that this error component is random, sometimes adding to the true score and sometimes diminishing it. We can never see the true score, only the observed score.

When we select a group because of its extreme scores (either very high or very low), we are including two types of persons: (1) those whose true scores are extreme and (2) those whose true scores do *not* fall in the extreme range, but the error component added to the true score has placed them in the extreme region. Similarly, we have excluded persons whose true scores are extreme but whose observed scores are below the cut-off level. For example, let's assume that we're using a test with a mean of 50, and a score of 70 or more identifies the most extreme 2% of the sample, which is the group we want to include in our study. We've shown the true score plus or minus the error component for the 10 subjects whose observed scores are 70 and for a few of the other subjects (Figure 3-15). Thus we have biased our sample to include an overrepresentation of people who have error scores in the direction *away from* the mean. Because the error component is random, when these people are retested only half of them will have error scores away from the mean (keeping them in the extreme range), and half will have error scores that move the observed score closer to the mean. On the whole, the group average on the second testing will be closer to the mean than on the first testing.

Figure 3-15. True score ± error component for 10 subjects with observed scores greater than 70 and 4 subjects with observed scores less than 70.

In practical terms, this means that if we select a group of subjects because they appear abnormal on some test (i.e., their score differs from the mean) and do *nothing* to them, they will seem to improve (move closer to the mean) when they are retested. So if we had intervened, it would be impossible to know if the improvement was caused by us or simply by regression effects.

The magnitude of this effect is inversely related to the reliability of the test; the less reliable the test is, the greater the regression effect. The reason is that reliability expresses the relative contributions of the true score and the error scores so that an unreliable test has a large error component (see the discussion on reliability in Chapter 4).

Regression toward the mean can be minimized in two ways: (1) by increasing the reliability of the test and (2) by testing each subject at least twice and requiring all the tests to be extreme before he or she is included in the study. This is often done in hypertension trials, in which the person has to have three consecutive abnormal readings before being called hypertensive.

Age-Period-Cohort Effects

We are often interested in how some variable changes over time. For example, Figure 3-16 shows the prevalence of dementia among people 65 years of age and up. The news ain't good—the prevalence doubles every 5 years. There are three possible explanations for this, which go by the name of Age-Period-Cohort (APC) effects.

An **age** effect is fairly easy to explain—older people are more likely to have Alzheimer's disease and other dementing disorders than are younger

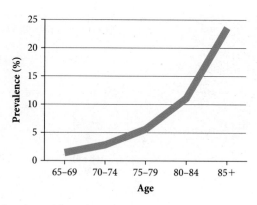

Figure 3-16. Prevalence of dementia as a function of age.

people. On the other hand, depression appears to peak in the mid-40s and then decrease with age. We see age effects with a variety of variables, such as height, vocabulary, and—at least among men—number of hair follicles (decreasing on the scalp, increasing in the ears). Most often, the relationship is monotonic, meaning that it steadily increases (or decreases), and perhaps reaches a plateau somewhere. In other cases, though, it can be more complex. As we've mentioned, depression seems to follow a ∩-shaped curve, and visits to the hospital are generally ∪-shaped: kids are often rushed to emergency rooms with cases of SPW (severe parental worry, a disorder that appears to occur only in first-born children), then visits drop in the teens and middle years, and rises again as our organs begin to fail, one after the other. Age effects are internal, in that they're due to physiological changes in the body, or to circumstances in a person's life, such as loss of social support as friends and relatives leave home or die.

With the variables we've mentioned so far, it's pretty obvious that age itself is the cause of the changes over time. But take a look at Figure 3-17, which shows the prevalence of psychological disorders in the last year for people 55 and over. The downward trend *could* be a function of age in that older people, for whatever reason, experience (or at least report) fewer problems than young whippersnappers (one of the few advantages of growing old; we can't think of many others, aside from the lack of peer pressure). But, the effect could also be due to cohort or period effects. A **cohort effect** is some external event that affects everyone born around the same time (an **age cohort**). For example, people who were in their 60s, 70s, and 80s when this survey was done in 2003 lived through two major influences: the Great Depression and World War II. There is some evidence that this may have led to greater psychological resilience, that protected these people from the effects of later adverse events. Similarly, people who experienced severe

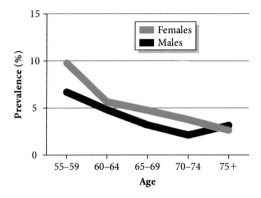

Figure 3-17. Prevalence of psychiatric disorders in the past year for men and women over the age of 55. (Modified from Streiner DL, Cairney J, Veldhuizen S: The epidemiology of psychological problems in the elderly, Can J Psychiatry 51: 185–191, 2006.)

malnutrition as infants due to crop failures or war suffer from life-long physical and intellectual sequelae.

The other possible explanation is a **period effect**; something that affects all people, irrespective of age. For example, Hurricane Katrina, which devastated New Orleans in 2007, resulted in many deaths, forced relocation to other cities, loss of jobs, and so on. So, period effects are similar to cohort effects in that they are due to external factors, but differ from them in that everyone is affected, not just the young.

The distinctions among these three effects sound pretty straightforward on paper, but in reality, they're hard to disentangle. No single study can determine whether the results are due to age, period, or cohort. It often requires a number of studies with people born at different times. The major problem in many studies, though, is trying to draw conclusions about longitudinal trends (i.e., age effects) from cross-sectional data. For example, studies done in the 1940s and 1950s tended to show a decline in intellectual ability that began fairly early in life. These studies were done by measuring the intelligence quotient (IQ) in a group of people in their teens, another group of people in their 20s, and so on. A different picture emerges when we follow one group of people over time, as we see in Figure 3-18. The cross-sectional data show the decline with time, but the longitudinal data show that inductive reasoning actually increases until we're ready for retirement, and then the decline is relatively slow and modest (we can now all breathe a sigh of relief). The problem with the earlier studies is that they confounded age with cohort; not only were the older subjects more advanced in years than the younger ones, but they were also exposed to a different educational and cultural environment, which accounted for most of the differences among the cohorts and hence for most of the apparent decline.

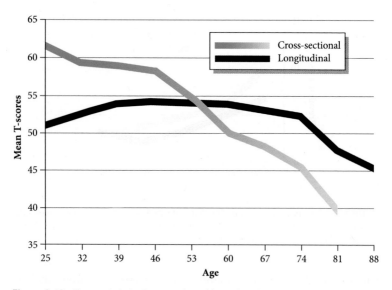

Figure 3-18. Changes in inductive reasoning with age based on longitudinal and cross-sectional data. (Modified from Schaie KW: The course of adult intellectual development, Am Psychol 49:304–313, 1994.)

Ecologic Fallacy

Ecologic studies attempt to demonstrate a relationship between two variables, such as suicide rate and religion, by using aggregate data. These are data about groups of people rather than individuals. For example, we can look at the rates of lung cancer per 100,000 individuals in a number of cities and see whether these are correlated with pollution levels.

Although this technique is inexpensive and has at times led to useful findings, there is one major problem—there is no guarantee that those people who developed lung cancer were the same ones who were exposed to the pollution. That is, it is possible (although unlikely) that pollution is unrelated to cancer of the lung but that pollution is caused by large factories. We know that cigarette smoking is related to social class and that factory workers smoke more heavily than the general population. So it may be that pollution is simply a marker for heavy smoking, and it is the smoking that is producing cancer.

The ecologic fallacy was nicely demonstrated by Robinson, who showed that there was a strong relationship ($r = 0.62$) between literacy rates and the proportion of nonnative born people; that is, regions with the largest number of immigrants had the lowest rates of illiteracy. Because most immigrants had relatively little education, especially in the 1930s when the data were collected, this seems to fly in the face of common sense. However, the individual correlation between literacy and foreign birth was -0.12, which is lower in magnitude (correlations based on individuals are almost always lower than ecologic correlations) and in the reverse direction.

The explanation is that immigrants usually settle in large cities, which have high rates of literacy, rather than in rural areas where literacy rates are lower. Thus *areas* with low rates of illiteracy have a high proportion of immigrants, but illiteracy and immigrant status are correlated (albeit weakly) within the *individual*.

RESEARCH STRATEGIES

The hallmark of a scientific theory is that its hypotheses are capable of being disproved. This does not always require experiments under the control of the researcher; astronomers haven't yet figured out how to experimentally induce stars to form or evolve. However, when experimental studies can be done, they can provide powerful tests of hypotheses that are not feasible when we have to rely solely on observations of naturally occurring events.

Over the years many different study designs have been developed to deal with the multitude of research questions that have been asked. We cannot begin to describe all of these methods here; entire books have been written on just this one area. Rather we have chosen the nine designs that are used most frequently. The first four (cross-sectional, ecologic, cohort, and case-control) are commonly referred to as **descriptive** or **analytic** designs. These are most appropriate when, for one reason or another, experimental control over the independent variable is not feasible. This would include, for instance, exposure to potentially harmful agents (e.g., cigarette smoke), situations in which there may be a long interval between exposure and outcome (e.g., diethylstilbestrol use and vaginal cancer in female offspring), or when our state of knowledge (or rather, ignorance) doesn't yet allow us to state whether there is an effect that's worth following up with a more expensive trial.

The second set of three designs are called **quasi-experimental**, and they cover a range of strategies where the researcher does not have complete control over all aspects of the study. These include the before-after study, the double-pretest design, and the interrupted time-series design. Very often, these designs take advantage of "experiments in nature;" that is, looking at the impact of events that have occurred naturally (e.g., rates of psychological depression following an economic one) or have been implemented by other people (e.g., whether death rates have decreased after changing the speed limit on highways or introducing motorcycle helmet laws). Some evaluators actually prefer these designs over true experiments, because what they may lack in terms of internal validity, they more than make up for with external validity—the interventions were actually carried out in the real world, and we don't have to worry about the biases affecting who gets into a study. We should note two things. First, there are other quasi-experimental designs that we're not going to describe, but if you're interested, read the bible by Shadish, Cook, and Campbell (see reference section). Second, the nomenclature gets a bit confusing, because various designs originated in different disciplines. What psychologists and educators, who were weaned on this book and its earlier incarnations, would call a *non-equivalent control group design*, people in the other health fields call a *cohort study*.

The last two designs (randomized control trial and cross-over) are called **experimental** because the intervention is under the control of the researcher. These methods are used (or should be used) in therapy trials because their results are least susceptible to the various threats to validity.

The important point is that the choice of study design depends on the question being asked. Usually several methods are possible, and we may look for the strongest (i.e., the one that allows the fewest alternative explanations for the results). However, we may instead opt for a "quick and dirty" design, even if it isn't the optimal one, simply to see if there is anything worth looking into at greater expense.

Nomenclature

Table 3-6 is based on the nomenclature introduced by Kleinbaum, Kupper, and Morgenstern and modified by the Department of Clinical Epidemiology and Biostatistics at McMaster University.

Table 3-6
Nomenclature for Epidemiologic Research Strategies

	Subject Allocation
N	Pool of eligible subjects
R	Random assignment
$\bar{R}$	Stratified random assignment

	Intervention
E	Exposure to intervention or causal factor
$\bar{E}$	Nonexposure
T	Treatment
$\bar{T}$	No treatment

	Outcome
--1 yr--	Follow-up (1-year)
C	Prevalent cases
$\bar{C}$	Noncase
D	Outcome present; incident case; or death
$\bar{D}$	Outcome not present; noncase; or survivor
O	Continuous outcome

Descriptive and Analytic Strategies

Cross-Sectional Survey

Design

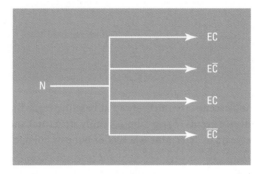

Example. A group of women (N) are interviewed to determine (1) whether they were sexually abused as children (E) and (2) if they now suffer from post-traumatic stress disorder (C).

Major Features. Exposure and caseness are determined simultaneously.

Advantages

1. This design is relatively inexpensive and simple to carry out, because no follow-up is required.
2. No one is exposed to the putative casual agent because of the study or denied a potentially beneficial therapy.
3. Loss to follow-up is not a problem.

Disadvantages

1. A cross-sectional design can establish association, but it is impossible to determine causation, because exposure and caseness are determined at the same time.
2. It is impossible to ensure that confounders are equally distributed among the groups.
3. Often either exposure or caseness or both depend upon recall, which is fallible.
4. This design is susceptible to the incidence-prevalence bias; that is, cases with early deaths and those in which evidence of exposure has disappeared are both missed.
5. The groups could end up having different sample sizes, resulting in a loss of statistical efficiency.
6. You cannot get estimates of incidence rates.

Descriptive and Analytic Strategies—cont´d

Longitudinal Survey
Design

$$EO\;\text{-----}|\;|\text{-----}\;C\;\text{-----}|\;|\text{-----}\;C$$

Example. Adolescents are interviewed at baseline regarding exposure to potentially adverse events (E; e.g., abuse, family structure) and then reassessed every few years to determine whether or not psychological problems later develop (C).

Major Features. The same people are re-interviewed on a periodic basis.

Advantages

1. With this design, it is possible to determine temporal relationship between exposure and outcome, yielding a stronger argument for causation.
2. It is possible to examine the natural history of a problem.
3. No one is exposed to the putative causal agent because of the study.

Disadvantages

1. It becomes progressively more difficult to keep the same people in the study as the number of follow-up interviews increases.
2. It is necessary to keep track of people as they move, change names, or die.
3. Even if the disorder was not detected at baseline, it does not necessarily mean that it was not present at a sub-clinical level, meaning that statements about temporal relationships and causality are still tentative.

Descriptive and Analytic Strategies—cont´d

Ecologic Study

Design

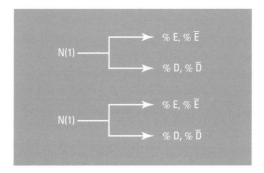

Example. Ecologic studies are used often in cancer research, in which the rates of cancer of different organs are examined by geographic area (county, province, or state). This has led to some fruitful hypotheses regarding the association between cancer of the esophagus and diet in Eastern Europe and China, for instance.

Major Features. The unit of analysis can be either a group (often defined geographically or on the basis of demographic variables) or time (e.g., mortality rate from measles from 1900 to 1960). The data are most often readily available.

Advantage

1. Data are usually available so this type of study is inexpensive.

Disadvantages

1. We know how many people were exposed within each group and how many have the outcome but *not* how many exposed people have the outcome; that is, it is possible that the outcome occurred in unexposed people and the variables are not related (see the discussion in *Threats to Validity* on ecologic fallacy earlier in this chapter).

2. Correlations from ecologic studies are usually much higher than in studies where both variables are gathered on the same individuals.

Descriptive and Analytic Strategies—cont′d

Cohort Study
Design

Example. A group of people who live in homes insulated with urea foam formaldehyde (UFFI) and a second group who did not live in UFFI homes are followed to determine the rates of upper respiratory tract infections, allergic reactions, and dermatological problems.

Major Features. Exposure to the putative casual agent or treatment is *not* under the researcher's control. Subjects are divided into exposed (or treated) and nonexposed (or untreated) groups on the basis of history. The design can be prospective (following the groups forward in time from the present) or retrospective (choosing groups that were formed some time in the past, and then following them forward from that time to the present).

Advantages
1. Treatment is not withheld from subjects, and they are not artificially subjected to potential hazards.
2. Subjects can be matched for possible confounders.
3. When the design is prospective, eligibility criteria and outcome assessments can be standardized.
4. It is administratively easier and less costly than randomized controlled trial (RCT).
5. It can establish the timing and directionality of events.
6. It can look at many outcomes following exposure.
7. It reduces the risk of survivor bias (i.e., non-inclusion of those who die early from the exposure).

Disadvantages
1. It may be difficult to obtain controls if therapy is popular or if most people have been exposed.
2. Exposure may be related to some other unknown factor that is correlated with the outcome (confounding).
3. Blindness among subjects and assessors may be difficult to achieve.
4. It is expensive to do well.
5. It may violate some statistical tests based on the assumption of randomization.

6. For rare disorders, large sample sizes or follow-up periods are necessary.
7. For long-term exposures (e.g., smoking, oral contraceptives), it may be difficult to quantify exposures that change over time.

Descriptive and Analytic Strategies—cont´d

Nested Case-Control Study
Design

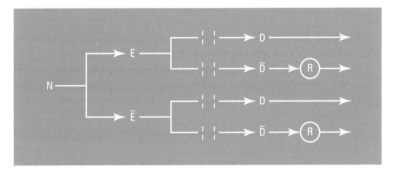

Example. Patients exposed to helicobacter pylori as children and controls are followed to determine who develops gastric ulcers. Blood is then drawn from all those who do (cases) and a random sample of those who do not develop ulcers to look at IgG antibodies against h. pylori.

Major Features. A case-control study is embedded within a cohort study.

Advantages
1. Expensive assays or invasive tests do not have to be run on everyone in the two cohorts.
2. A very efficient design when the prevalence of the outcome is low.
3. Better control over potential confounders through matching than in a case-control study.
4. Controls are from the same population as the cases.

Disadvantages
1. As always, matching on key characteristics is important.
2. Some loss of statistical efficiency because the full cohort is not analyzed.

Quasi-Experimental Designs

Before-After Studies
Design

$$O_1 \qquad E \qquad O_2$$

Example. Rates of falls in a long-term care facility are compared before (O_1) and after (O_2) the introduction of a falls-prevention program (E).

Major Features. This design is often used when the intervention is not under the researcher's control, and there are no comparable comparison groups.

Advantages
1. The intervention is often a "natural experiment," so there is little concern that it can be implemented.
2. It is usually cheap and fast, and may use data collected for other purposes.
3. It may be the only feasible design to study the effects of natural events.

Disadvantages
1. It is impossible to know whether anything else was going on at the same time that may have led to the change.
2. Scores may change simply because of maturational effects.

Quasi-Experimental Designs

Removed-Treatment (A–B–A) Study
Design

Example. Hospitalization rates are measured before (O_1) and after (O_2) family physicians are paid a bonus for reducing the number of their patients referred to hospital (T). Rates are measured again before (O_3) and after (O_4) the bonus plan is stopped.

Major Features. The intervention can be implemented and removed any number of times. This can also be done with individual patients using an active treatment and a placebo. In behavioral psychology, it is called an A-B-A design, with A indicating no (or sham) treatment, and B indicating the active treatment.

Advantages
1. It may be the only feasible design when even non-equivalent control groups cannot be obtained.
2. The validity of the conclusion is strengthened each time this pattern is repeated.(e.g., A-B-A-B-A).
3. When a placebo condition is used, the order of treatment and non-treatment can be random.

Disadvantages
1. It cannot be used if the effect of the treatment is long-lasting.
2. It may be ethically questionable to remove a treatment that works.
3. There may be resentment if it is noticed that the intervention is removed.
4. There may be threats to validity from maturation and/or history.

Quasi-Experimental Designs—cont´d

Double-Pretest Design (Non-Equivalent Control Group)
Design

$$O_{A1} \qquad E \qquad O_{A2}$$
$$O_{B1} \qquad\qquad O_{B2}$$

Example. Caesarian-section rates are compared before (O_{A1}) and after (O_{A2}) an intervention (E) to encourage vaginal births among women who have had previous C-sections. Rates are also compared for first-time mothers (O_{B1} and O_{B2}).

Major Features. Outcome A should be affected by the intervention; outcome B should not be, but should change only if there were overall changes in the organization or people.

Advantages

1. The intervention is often a "natural experiment," so there is little concern that it can be implemented.
2. It is usually cheap and fast, and may use data collected for other purposes.
3. The second outcome measure determines, to some degree, if there were other factors, such as maturation or organizational changes, that may have occurred at the same time.
4. It may be the only feasible design to study the effects of natural events.

Disadvantages

1. It is impossible to know if anything else was going on at the same time that may have led to changes in both outcome measures.
2. It may be difficult to find the second outcome measure.

Quasi-Experimental Designs—cont´d

Interrupted Time Series Design
Design

$$O_{B1} \quad O_{B2} \quad O_{B3} \quad \cdots \quad O_{Bj} \quad E \quad O_{A1} \quad O_{A2} \quad O_{A3} \quad \cdots \quad O_{Ak}$$

Example. The number of patients with *C. difficile* is measured every month before (O_{B1} through O_{Bj}) and after (O_{A1} through O_{Ak}) a hand-washing educational program (E).

Major Features. Having many measures over time allows us to see whether there were any trends before the intervention that could have simply continued after it was implemented. It also reduces (but does not eliminate) the influence of external factors accounting for the difference. The number of observations before and after the intervention do not have to be the same.

Advantages
1. The intervention is often a "natural experiment," so there is little concern that it can be implemented.
2. It is usually cheap and fast, and may use data collected for other purposes.
3. It allows us to determine if the intervention led to a change in the slope of the line, its level, or both.

Disadvantages
1. It is still possible that other events could have led to the change.
2. Many (ideally, at least 15) measures are required before and after the intervention to be confident about the slopes and levels of the pre- and post-intervention lines.
3. It may not be possible to gather enough data points, especially after the intervention, before an answer is required.

Quasi-Experimental Designs—cont´d

Case Control Study

Design

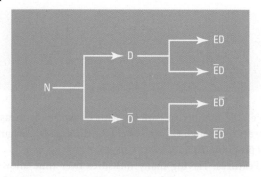

Example. The mothers of children born with (D) and without ($\overline{D}$) neural tube defects are interviewed to determine whether they took folate during their pregnancy.

Major Features. The groups are identified on the basis of the *outcome* (e.g., birth defects), and the search for exposure (to folic acid) is retrospective.

Advantages

1. It can be done relatively quickly and inexpensively.
2. It may be the only feasible method for rare disorders or for situations in which there is a long lag between exposure and outcome.
3. It usually requires fewer subjects than cross-sectional studies.

Disadvantages

1. It relies on recall or records to determine exposure, and both are notoriously inaccurate.
2. The groups may be confounded; that is, exposure may have been caused by some other factor that is correlated with the outcome (e.g., income, area of residence, age).
3. It may be difficult to select and then find an appropriate control group.
4. If the index group is aware of the hypothesis, there is the possibility of recall bias.

Experimental Designs

Randomized Controlled Trial

Design

Example. Hemiplegic stroke patients currently receiving physiotherapy are randomly assigned to receive or not receive transcutaneous stimulation. After 3 months, they are compared on walking speed (continuous outcome) and presence or absence of footdrop (discrete outcome).

Major Features. Subject allocation to treatments or exposure is under the control of the experimenter.

Advantages

1. Groups are likely more comparable because confounding variables are probably balanced.
2. There is a greater likelihood that patients, staff, and assessors can be blinded.
3. Most statistical tests rest on the assumption of random allocation.

Disadvantages

1. These trials are expensive in terms of time and money.
2. Those who volunteer may not be representative of all patients.
3. A potentially effective treatment is withheld from some subjects, or some may be exposed to a possibly dangerous one.
4. Final results may not be available for many years.
5. It assumes participants actually did or did not get the intervention as planned (i.e., total adherence in the treatment group, and no contamination within the comparison group).
6. It also assumes very low attrition, and the reasons for drop-out are unrelated to the treatment (or lack of it).

Experimental Designs—cont´d

Cross-Over Design
Design

Example. Patients are randomly allocated to receive carbamazepine to control their manic-depressive disorder or a placebo. After 4 weeks they are given a placebo until all the drug is out of their system. Then those who had been given carbamazepine are given placebo for 4 weeks, and those given placebo are given the active drug.

Major Features. Randomization is under the researcher's control; all patients receive both the active treatment and the placebo (or control treatment).

Advantages

1. Subjects serve as their own controls, thereby reducing error variance. Consequently, fewer subjects generally are needed than for RCTs.
2. All subjects receive the treatment at least for some period.
3. Statistical tests assuming randomization can be used.
4. Blindness of patients, staff, and assessors can be maintained.

Disadvantages

1. Subjects who responded to the treatment are taken off it and given placebo (or the alternative treatment).
2. The wash-out period with some drugs can be lengthy, during which time the patients are often given placebos.
3. It cannot be used if the treatment has any permanent effects (e.g., educational programs, physiotherapy, behavior therapy).

META-ANALYSIS

In some areas, it appears as if the problem is not that there are no studies, but rather that there are too many, often with contradictory findings. **Meta-analysis** is a method of combining the results of two or more studies in order to arrive at an overall estimate of the magnitude of the effect of an intervention. Since its introduction in 1977, with Smith and Glass's meta-analysis of psychotherapy trials, there has been an exponential growth in the number published each year. The key elements of a meta-analysis are:

The Question. The question should be as specific as possible. One that asks, "Does radiotherapy work for breast cancer?" will return hundreds of articles, most of which will be irrelevant. A tighter one, like, "Does radiotherapy, following lumpectomy, improve the five-year survival rate in women with Stage II breast cancer," specifies (a) the treatment, (b) the target group, and (c) the outcome of interest. However, if the question is too narrow, then there may be very few studies.

The Criteria. Criteria for including an article in a meta-analysis must be spelled out *before* a literature search is done; and must *not* include the outcome (positive or negative) as a criterion. The criteria are usually based on the design (e.g., only RCTs; RCTs plus cohort studies; etc.) and issues of internal and external validity (e.g., proportion of patients followed up; length or intensity of the treatment). Ideally, two raters assess each article, in order to evaluate the reliability of the selection process.

The Search. The search should be as thorough as possible. This would include computerized databases, such as MEDLINE, PsycLit, CINAHL, Cancerlit; checking the references of retrieved articles to see what may have been missed; and contacting experts in the field. There is some controversy regarding whether unpublished papers (the "gray literature") should be

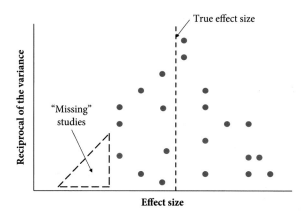

Figure 3-19.   A funnel plot, showing the effect size for each study. Publication bias is evident by the lack of studies in the dotted triangle.

included. Those who argue in favor say that there is a bias against publishing studies with negative findings, so limiting the review to only published papers overestimates the actual effectiveness of the intervention. Those arguing against say that the gray literature is not peer reviewed, and that any well-done study will be published eventually, even if the results are negative. It's probably best to include unpublished articles, and then run the meta-analysis twice: once with them included, and again excluding them. If the results are similar, no problem; if they differ, then the findings must be interpreted with caution.

A larger issue is what to do with regard to methodological quality. Some authors go to enormous pains to screen out poor-quality articles; others, including Glass, the father of meta-analysis, "take all comers." While it would seem that quality would indeed affect the outcome, it is a little less evident, on closer inspection, just *how* it would affect it. In the health sciences literature, it is generally assumed that poor studies lead to large treatment effects, and that, when good studies are done later, the effects disappear. That may be so. If, for example, patients or caregivers were unblinded, this might lead to a bigger effect. On the other hand, poor studies might result in poorer compliance, poorer follow-up, and so on, all of which would dilute the treatment effect. The relation between quality and treatment effect has been looked at a number of times, and the results are indeed mixed, with some studies showing no relation, some showing that good quality leads to smaller effects, and occasional studies showing the opposite. Interestingly, the "mother of all reviews," a true systematic review of systematic reviews,

Figure 3-20. A forest plot.

involving 302 systematic reviews including roughly 14,000 articles, showed no relation between study quality and effect size, as long as there was some kind of contemporaneous control group, and no relation between randomization and effect size. Apropos our earlier comment, there was, however, a large publication bias.

Abstracting the Findings. Each article is abstracted; the relevant information includes (as a minimum) the magnitude of the difference, the sample size, and anything else that may influence the results, such as the setting (tertiary care teaching hospital vs. community hospital), dosage, length of treatment, and so on. Ideally, this will also be done independently by two raters to check for accuracy.

Looking for Problems. There are (at least) two major problems that can arise. First, as we mentioned, there is the well-documented bias against submitting and publishing negative findings (at least in journals published in English; it's always possible to get them published in a journal published in Urdu or Pashto). This is also referred to as the "file drawer" problem, since these unloved and unwanted studies languish in the bottom of researchers' file drawers. We usually look for publication bias with a *funnel plot*. This is a graph, like the one in Figure 3-19, where the X-axis is the effect size, and the Y-axis is the sample size (or the reciprocal of the variance, which boils down to the same thing). If there is no bias, then the graph should look like an upside-down funnel. If there's bias, then usually the lower left corner is truncated; the dots that are missing from the triangle are likely articles that never got published. The second problem is *heterogeneity of results*, which means that the effect sizes vary considerably from one study to the next. There are various mathematical tests for this, but there is also much debate what to do if it's found. Some people advocate dropping the outlying studies, since they're "obviously" studying something else. Others (including ourselves) say to keep them in, and then look for the possible reasons for heterogeneity.

Combining Results. At this point, each study has been reduced to an effect size—an odds ratio, a relative risk, a standardized mean difference, or whatever (these will be discussed in the next chapter). We could simply add them up and get the average, but this ignores one major issue: not all studies are created equal. One with a very large sample size should be given more weight than a small trial. We handle this by weighting each effect size by either the sample size or the reciprocal of the variance—bigger trials, or those with less variability in their findings, carry more weight.

Reporting Results. At the end, what we have is a mean, weighted effect size. Often, though, we go a bit further. First, we can display the results for each study in a *forest plot* such as in Figure 3-20. Looking at it, can you see why it's called a forest plot? Neither can we. Each study is a separate line. The box indicates the effect size, and the area of the box is proportional to the sample size—bigger study, bigger box. The lines show the 95% confidence interval; if the line crosses the vertical dotted line, which represents no effect of the intervention, then that trial did not have statistically significant results. The diamond at the bottom shows the overall weighted effect size. In this case, although five of the nine studies weren't significant, the combined effect was that the treatment worked. Finally, we can try to determine why some studies had large effect sizes and others small ones: was it the setting, the dosage, the methodological rigor, or something else?

Truth. Because meta-analyses are supposedly objective analyses based on a thorough literature search, can we be assured that the results represent "truth"? Unfortunately, no. Because there are so many steps in the process, with judgment calls required at each one of them, it is very disconcerting, but not that unusual, to find meta-analyses in the same area coming to different conclusions. The reader's guiding motto must be *caveat emptor*.

C.R.A.P. DETECTORS

C.R.A.P. Detector III-1

Question. In one of the seminal books on the etiology of homosexuality, Bieber and his associates derived their sample by mailing three copies of a questionnaire to fellow members of a New York–based psychoanalytic society. The analysts filled them out for any homosexual patient they had in therapy. If the psychiatrist had fewer than three such patients in treatment, he or she was to fill out the remaining questionnaires on male heterosexual patients; the heterosexual subjects constituted the control group. What are the problems with this sampling strategy?

Answer. Unfortunately, a listing of all the problems would fill a book thicker than this one. First, persons who elect to go into psychoanalysis are not representative of the general population. Obviously, those who are happy with their lives never spend time on the analytic couch. Second, those who are unhappy but poor must settle for less comfortable and less expensive chairs or get no help at all. Finally, leaving the choice of which patients to include up to the individual analysts opens the door to a host of biases; it is doubtful whether the sample would include patients who didn't improve or who didn't match the psychoanalytic sample.

C.R.A.P. Detector III-2

Question. Those who disapprove of social assistance programs state that welfare fosters dependence and encourages people to behave in ways that enable them to remain on assistance for a long time. The opponents buttress their arguments with surveys showing that, at any one time, the majority of welfare recipients have been on it for extended periods. How much can we trust these data?

Answer. This is a nice example of the incidence-prevalence bias. Figure 3-21, *A*, shows the proportion of women who have ever received Aid for Families with Dependent Children (AFDC) and how long they were on it. Of these women, 30 percentage were on AFDC for only 1 or 2 years, and 70 percentage received it for less than 8 years. However, if the investigators had done a cross-sectional survey that asked women currently on AFDC how long they had been on it, a different picture would emerge. Now, as Figure 3-21, *B*, shows, the vast majority (65 percentage) have been getting benefits for more than 7 years. The problem is that long-term recipients are more likely to be picked up in a one-time survey than short-term recipients who had been on AFDC in the past but were not at the time of the survey.

Percent of women who have ever received AFDC

Percent of women receiving AFDC at a particular time

Figure 3-21. A, Percentage of women who have ever received Aid for Families with Dependent Children (AFDC) and length of time they received it. **B,** Percentage of women who received AFDC at a particular time and the length of time they had been receiving it. (From Duncan GJ, Hill MS, Hoffman SD: Welfare dependence within and across generations, *Science* 239:467–471,1988.)

C.R.A.P. Detector III-3

Question. Schroeder, among others, concluded that there was a relationship between water hardness and cardiovascular disease. Specifically, he found a correlation of –0.56, which indicated that states with the softest water had the highest death rate for heart disease. Should you be worried if you live in an area with soft water?

Answer. Schroeder's study used data aggregated at the level of states, and as such it was susceptible to the ecologic fallacy. Comstock followed up this finding by gathering data on individuals and found no relationship between cardiovascular disease and trace elements in water. So what holds at the level of the community or state may not obtain for the individual.

C.R.A.P. Detector III-4

Question. According to Ederer the 10 top batters in the American League in 1968 had a mean batting average of .414, and the 10 worst batted an average of .083 in the first week of play. As can be seen in Figure 3-22, by the second week both groups were batting in the low .200s. Does this mean that the good batters suddenly got worse and the bad batters mysteriously got better?

Answer. This is an example of the regression toward the mean effect. On the average, persons chosen because they are above the mean on one occasion tend to "regress" down toward it at a second measurement period, and those below the mean regress upward. Ederer showed the same effect with serum cholesterol (Figure 3-23): the higher the baseline level, the greater the later "improvement," whether the subjects had been on a cholesterol-lowering diet or a control diet.

Figure 3-22. Mean batting average of 10 best and 10 worst batters.

Figure 3-23. Example of regression toward the mean effect: the higher the baseline serum cholesterol level, the greater the subsequent improvement, regardless of diet. (From Schroeder HA: Relationship between mortality from cardiovascular disease and treated water supplies: variations in states and 163 largest municipalities of the United States, JAMA 172:1902–1908, 1960.)

REFERENCES

Sadetzki S, Chetrit A, Jarus-Hakak A, et al.: Cellular phone use and risk of benign and malignant parotid gland tumors—a nationwide case-control study, *Am J Epidemiol* 167:457–467, 2008.

Schüz J, Jacobsen R, Olsen JH, et al.: Cellular telephone use and cancer risk: an update of a nationwide Danish cohort, *J Natl Cancer Inst* 98:1707–1713, 2006.

Yet Some More History

Chadwick E: *Report of an enquiry into the sanitary conditions of the labouring population of Great Britain*, London, 1842, Poor Law *Commission.*

Chenier NM: *Reproductive hazards at work*, Ottawa, 1982, Canadian Advisory Council on the Status of Women.

Department of Health and Social Security: *Inequalities in health: report of a working group chaired by Sir Douglas Black*, London, 1980, DHSS.

Kemp P, editor: *The Oxford companion to ships and the sea*, Oxford, 1988, Oxford University Press.

Lilienfeld AM: *Foundations of epidemiology*, New York, 1976, Oxford University Press.

Lind J: *A treatise of the scurvey*, Edinburgh, 1753, Sands, Murray, and Cochrane.

Marmot MG, Smith GD, Stansfeld S, et al.: Health inequalities among British civil servants: the Whitehall II study, *The Lancet* 337:1387–93, 1991.

Streiner DL, Cairney J: The social science contribution to psychiatric epidemiology. In Cairney J, Streiner DL, editors: *Mental disorder in Canada: An epidemiological perspective*, Toronto, 2010, University of Toronto Press.

Trachtman P: Hero for our time. *Smithsonian* 34–41, Jan. 2002.

Voltaire: *Letters on the English or lettres philosophiques*, Whitefish, Mont., 2004, Kessinger Publishing.

106   PDQ EVIDENCE-BASED PRINCIPLES AND PRACTICE

Design Elements

Number of Observations
Bagby RM, Silverman I, Ryan DP: Effects of mental health legislative reforms in Ontario, *Can Psychol* 28:21–29, 1987.

Comparison Groups
Hill AB: *Statistical methods in clinical and preventive medicine*, Edinburgh, 1962, Livingstone.

Hinshaw HC, Feldman WH, Pfuetze KH: Treatment of tuberculosis with streptomycin: summary of observations on 100 cases, *JAMA* 132:778–782, 1946.

Whom to Count
Norman GR, Streiner DL: *Biostatistics: the bare essentials*, 3rd edition, Toronto, 2007, PMPH-USA.

Streiner DL: The two Es of research: efficacy and effectiveness trials, *Can J Psychiatry* 47:347–351, 2002.

Sampling

Cluster Sampling
Donner A, Birkett N, Buck C: Randomization by cluster: sample size requirements and analysis, *Am J Epidemiol* 114:906–914, 1981.

Spitzer WO, Sackett DL, Sibley JC: The Burlington randomized trial of the nurse practitioner, *N Engl J Med* 290:251–256, 1974.

Haphazard Sampling
Mueller PS, Watkin DM: Plasma unesterified fatty acid concentrations in neoplastic disease, *J Lab Clin Med* 57:95–108, 1961.

Quick AJ: Hemolysate prothrombin consumption time: a new test for thromboplastinogenic coagulation defects, *J Lab Clin Med* 57:290–299, 1961.

Subject Allocation

Random Allocation
Schultz KF, Grimes DA: Generation of allocation sequences in randomised trials: chance, not choice, *Lancet* 359:515–519, 2002.

Minimization
Altman DG, Bland JM: Treatment allocation by minimisation, *BMJ* 330:843, 2005.

Scott NW, McPherson GC, Ramsay CR, Campbell MK: The method of minimization for allocation to clinical trials: a review, *Control Clin Trials* 23:662–674, 2002.

Taves, DR: Minimization: a new method of assigning patients to treatment and control groups, *Clin Pharm Ther* 15:443–453, 1974.

Other Forms of Randomization

Jadad A: *Randomised controlled trials*, London, BMJ Books, 1998.

Rosenberger, WF, Lachin, JM. The use of response-adaptive designs in clinical trials, *Control Clin Trials* 14:471–484, 1993.

Zelen M: Play the winner rule and the controlled clinical trial, *J Am Stat Assoc* 64:131–146,1969.

Zelen M: A new design for randomized clinical trials, *N Engl J Med* 300:1242–1245, 1979.

Threats to Validity

Cook, TD, Campbell DT: *Quasi-experimentation: design issues for field settings*, Chicago, 1979, Rand McNally.

Subject Selection Biases

Sackett DL: Bias in analytic research, *J Chronic Dis* 32:51–63, 1979.

Healthy Worker Bias

Seltzer CC, Jablon S: Effects of selection on mortality, *Am J Epidemiol* 100:367–372, 1974.

Incidence-Prevalence Bias

American Psychiatric Association: *Diagnostic and statistical manual of mental disorders, fourth edition, text revision*, Washington DC, 2000, APA.

Harding CM, Zubin J, Strauss JS: Chronicity in schizophrenia: fact, partial fact, or artifact? *Hosp Community Psychiatry* 38:477–486, 1987.

Berkson's Bias

Maric N, Myin-Germeys I, Delespaul P, de Graff R, Vollebergh W, Van Os J: Is our concept of schizophrenia influenced by Berkson's bias? *Soc Psychiatry Psychiatr Epidemiol* 39:600–605, 2004.

Volunteer Bias

American Heart Association: *The national diet-heart study: final report. American Heart Association Monograph No. 18*, New York, 1980, AHA.

Horwitz RI, Horwitz SM: Adherence to treatment and health outcomes, *Arch Intern Med* 153:1863–1868, 1993.

Coronary Drug Project Research Group: Influence of adherence to treatment and response to cholesterol on mortality in the coronary drug project, *N Engl J Med* 303:1038–1041, 1980.

Sims ACP: Importance of a high tracing-rate in long-term medical follow-up studies, *Lancet* ii:433–435, 1973.

Hawthorne Effect

Bramel D, Friend R: Hawthorne, the myth of the docile worker, and class bias in psychology, *Am Psychol* 36:867–878, 1981.

Frank JD: *Persuasion and healing*, Baltimore, 1961, Johns Hopkins Press. Parsons HM: What happened at Hawthorne? *Science* 183:922–932, 1974.

Blinding

Balon J, Aker PD, Crowther ER, Danielson C, Cox PG, O'Shaughnessy D, Walker C, Goldsmith CH, Duku E, Sears MR: A comparison of active and simulated chiropractic manipulation as adjunctive treatment for childhood asthma. *N Engl J Med* 339:1013–1020, 1998.

Beecher HK: The powerful placebo, *JAMA* 159:1602–1606, 1955.

Rosenthal R: *Experimenter effects in behavioral research*, New York, 1966 Appleton-Century-Crofts.

Proxy Measures

Surrogate End Points

Furberg CD, Psaty, BM, Meyer JV: Nifedipine: dose-related increase in mortality in patients with coronary heart disease, *Circulation* 92:1326–1331, 1995.

Kessler DA, Feiden KL: Faster evaluation of vital drugs, *Sci Am* 272(3):48–54, 1995.

Strandberg TE, Salomaa VV, Naukkarinen VA: Long-term mortality after 5-year multifactorial primary prevention of cardiovascular diseases in middle-aged men, *JAMA* 266:1225–1229, 1991.

Recall Bias

Cannell CF, Fisher G, Bakker T: Reporting on hospitalization in the Health Interview Survey, *Vital Health Stat 3*, No. 6. Hyattsville, Public Health Service, 1965.

Rockenbauer M, Olsen J, Czeizel A, Pedersen L, Sorensen H, EuroMAP Group: Recall bias in a case-control surveillance system on the use of medicine during pregnancy, *Epidemiology* 12:461–466, 2001.

Confounding

Hennekens CH, Buring JE: *Epidemiology in medicine*, Boston, 1987, Little, Brown.

Interactions

Shapiro S, Slone D, Rosenberg L: Oral-contraceptive use in relation to myocardial infarction, *Lancet* i:743–746, 1979.

Age-Period-Cohort Effects

Elder GH. *Children of the great depression: social change in life experience*, Chicago, 1974, University of Chicago Press.

Jorm AF, Korten AE, Henderson AS: The prevalence of dementia: a quantitative integration of the literature, *Acta Psychiatr Scand* 76:465–479, 1987.

Horn JL, Donaldson G: On the myth of intellectual decline in adulthood, *Am Psychol* 31:701–719, 1976.

Konczacki ZA. Infant mal-nutrition in sub-Saharan Africa: a problem in socio-economic development, *Can J Afr Stud* 6:433–449, 1972.

Schaie KW: The course of adult intellectual development, *Am Psychol* 49:304–313,1994.

Streiner DL, Cairney J, Veldhuizen S: The epidemiology of psychological problems in the elderly. *Can J Psychiatry* 51:185–191, 2006.

Ecologic Fallacy

Robinson WS: Ecological correlations and the behavior of individuals, *Am Sociol Rev* 15:351–357, 1950.

Research Strategies

Nomenclature

Kleinbaum DG, Kupper LL, Morgenstern H: *Epidemiologic research: principles and quantitative methods*, Belmont, Calif., 1982, Lifetime Learning Publications.

Shadish WR, Cook TD, Campbell DT: *Experimental and quasi-experimental designs for generalized causal inference*, Boston, 2002, Houghton Mifflin.

Case-Control Study

Schulz KF, Grimes DA: Case-control studies: research in reverse, *Lancet* 359:431–434, 2002.

Cohort Study

Grimes DA, Schulz KF: Cohort studies: marching towards outcome, *Lancet* 359:341–345, 2002.

Nested Case Control Study

Lin JT, Wang LY, Wang JT, Wang TH, Yang CS, Chen CJ: A nested case-control study on the association between Helicobacter pylori infection and gastric cancer risk in a cohort of 9775 men in Taiwan, *Anticancer Res* 15:603–606, 1995.

Meta-Analysis

Dickersin K: The existence of publication bias and risk factors for its occurrence. *JAMA* 263:1385–1359, 1990.

Lipsey MW, Wilson DB: The efficacy of psychological, educational, and behavioral treatment: confirmation from meta-analysis. *Am Psychol* 48:1181–1209, 1993.

Rosenthal R: The file drawer problem and tolerance for null results, *Psychol Bull* 86:638–641, 1979.

Smith ML, Glass GV: Meta-analysis of psychotherapy outcome studies, *Am Psychol* 32:752–760, 1977.

C.R.A.P. Detectors

Bieber I, Dain HJ, Dince PR: *Homosexuality*, New York, 1962, Basic Books.

Comstock GW: Fatal arteriosclerotic heart disease, water hardness at home, and socioeconomic characteristics, *Am J Epidemiol* 94:1–10, 1971.

Duncan GJ, Hill MS, Hoffman SD: Welfare dependence within and across generations, *Science* 239:467–471, 1988.

Ederer F: Serum cholesterol changes: effects of diet and regression toward the mean, *J Chronic Dis* 25:277–289, 1972.

Schroeder HA: Relationship between mortality from cardiovascular disease and treated water supplies: variations in states and 163 largest municipalities of the United States, *JAMA* 172:1902–1908, 1960.

Sampling

Abramson JH: *Survey methods in community medicine*, Edinburgh, 1974, Churchill-Livingstone.

Levy P, Lemeshow S: *Sampling for health professionals*, Belmone, Calif., 1980, Lifetime Learning Publications.

Subject Allocation

Hoel DG, Sobel M, Weiss GH: A survey of adaptive sampling for clinical trails. In Elashoff RM, editor: *Perspectives in biometrics*, vol 1, New York, 1975, Academic Press.

Threats to Validity

Ederer F: Patient bias, investigator bias and the double-masked procedure in clinical trials, *Am J Med* 58:295–299, 1975.

Morgenstern H: Uses of ecologic analysis in epidemiological research, *Am J Public Health* 72:1336–1344, 1982.

Rosenthal R, Rosnow RL: *The volunteer subject*, New York, 1975, Wiley.

Sackett DL: Bias in analytic research, *J Chronic Dis* 32:51–63, 1979.

Walter SD: Cause-deleted proportional mortality analysis and the healthy worker effect, *Stat Med* 5:61–71, 1986.

Yang Y: Age-period-cohort distinctions. In Markides KS, editor: *Encyclopedia of health and aging*, Thousand Oaks, Calif., 2007, Sage.

Epidemiologic Research Strategies

Cook TD, Campbell DT: *Quasi-experimentation: design issues for field settings*, Chicago, 1979, Rand McNally.

Kleinbaum DG, Kupper LL, Morgenstern H: *Epidemiologic research: principles and quantitative methods*, Belmont, Calif., 1982, Lifetime Learning Publications.

Schlesselman JJ: *Case-control studies: design, conduct, analysis*, New York, 1982, Oxford University Press.

4

Measurement

We live in a cancer-phobic society. For several decades the person on the street has been bombarded with the carcinogen of the week to the point of numbing exhaustion. This epidemic reached ludicrous limits when it was announced, in all seriousness, that mother's milk "caused" cancer because it contained trace amounts of polychlorinated biphenyl (PCB) and other awful chemicals and that children should be breast-fed for a maximum of 6 months because of this "hazard."

In part, the present dilemma can be laid at the feet of zealous legislators and news-hungry media folks; in part, the problem exists simply because our technical expertise has far outstripped our legislative apparatus. Laws about cancer in the environment were passed several decades ago when the prevailing attitude was that any amount of a carcinogen in the soil, air, or water was too much. Since that time, technical improvements in analytic instrumentation have allowed us to detect trace amounts of chemicals that are orders of magnitude smaller than the amounts detectable when the laws were passed (literally equivalent to a martini made with a drop of vermouth in a swimming pool of gin). However, the laws remain on the books, and any attempt to repeal them at this stage would promote a rapid demise to any political career.

In part, too, the issue is epidemiologic. Epidemiologists, oncologists, and toxicologists tend to view the issue of causation as a binary variable—either something causes cancer or it doesn't. Admittedly, some attempt is made to quantify the risk by extrapolation from animal data to humans. Nevertheless, it would certainly assist the field, and perhaps our quality of life, if we would pause to ask just how much cancer a particular agent might cause. Of course, this question demands some means of quantifying the degree of risk to life and limb from a particular agent.

This chapter deals explicitly with this issue, discussing a variety of **measures of association** used by epidemiologists. The problems to which these measures can be applied are far-ranging, from the estimation of the risk to health from an environmental agent, to the benefit of treatment, the agreement between a diagnostic test and a "gold standard," and issues of observer agreement.

ISSUES IN CHOOSING A MEASURE

The issue of measurement is critical to much of science. Lord Kelvin, a distinguished physicist of the 1800s, once said:

> I often say that when you can measure what you are speaking about, and express it in numbers, you know something about it; but when you cannot express it in numbers, your knowledge is of a meager and unsatisfactory kind; it may be the beginning of knowledge, but you have scarcely, in your thoughts, advanced to the stage of science whatever the matter may be.

Epidemiology is not immune to these admonitions. The issue of measurement in many sciences is, by and large, a technical issue of instrumentation and of developing the right bit of apparatus to measure some phenomenon with the appropriate degree of precision. In epidemiology the issues are a bit more conceptual, and much thought must be directed to the appropriate selection of which variable to measure in the first place. Often the choice of variable represents a deliberate compromise; for example, in looking at the effects of an educational strategy for practicing physicians, one could decide to measure the increase in knowledge of the participants, a variable that is likely sensitive to the educational strategy and can be easily tested with methods like multiple-choice questions. Unfortunately, this choice begs the issue of whether the increased knowledge will be translated into a change in physician behavior with patients. In turn, we should worry whether the physician's admonitions will change patient behavior, whether this behavioral change will actually result in improved health, and whether the improvement in health will result in increased longevity or decreased morbidity. It is evident that the further we get from the intervention, the more socially relevant the outcomes are but the less likely they are to be sensitive to the intervention.

The Dimensions of Measurement

Epidemiologists have categorized the wide number of potential choices in the measurement of the effects of illness into the six Ds—death, disease, disability, discomfort, dissatisfaction, and debt. A little creativity can easily result in some additions to the list: psychiatrists would like to look at dysphoria and depression, and sociologists might examine disenfranchisement or dysfunction.

Some of these variables, like death and debt, are relatively easy to measure and hence are frequently used in studies in epidemiology. Others, like dissatisfaction and disability, are notoriously difficult to measure and have been the making of many a career in epidemiology. We will avoid, for the most part, the technical issues surrounding the measurement of these variables; the important point is that the Ds serve as a reminder that measurement of dependent variables or outcomes need not be confined to the traditional measures like death and disease.

The choice of an outcome variable is almost inevitably a compromise based on the interplay among the following factors.

Precision of Measurement

Measures that are subject to a large degree of random variation or individual interpretation are less useful than measures that are more precise. The judgment of precision cannot be made on an a priori basis; careful studies have shown appallingly high error rates in many areas of clinical medicine, such as radiology, that conventional wisdom would suggest are highly objective. Methods to assess precision are reviewed later in this section.

Logistical Factors

Measures are often chosen simply because they are inexpensive. Cost is certainly one criterion, as are other logistical factors like the likelihood of obtaining compliance or the ease of entering the data.

Ethical Issues

Some measurements are unsuitable for ethical reasons. No ethics committee would permit coronary angiography to be performed on all patients in a trial, regardless of cost, simply because of the risks associated with the procedure (unless the test was a part of the patients' regular care).

Importance

Often the most important variables, in terms of their burden on the affected individual, are the most impractical to use in studies. One good example is death. It has considerable importance to the individuals involved. However, although it is precise and easy to measure, death is often rejected as an outcome variable in studies because it occurs too infrequently (thank goodness), and thus the follow-up period required would be too long. As a result, investigators often substitute other variables that are less important but more available for measurement. As one example, hypoglycemic agents were adopted because they demonstrated the appropriate effect on blood sugar, which is much easier to measure than diabetes (although not as relevant). Much later, the widespread use of the drugs was discontinued because long-term studies showed that the lower blood sugar level had no impact on longevity or complications from the disease.

Sensitivity

For a variable to be useful, there must be some reasonable chance that it is related to, or likely to change with, the independent variable under study. As an example, researchers often select a laboratory test result as a measure of effect of a risk factor or therapeutic intervention. For instance, several studies have looked at the effect of formaldehyde on lower respiratory tract disease using measures of pulmonary function as the dependent variable. The choice is reasonable in some respects; pulmonary function can be measured with a high degree of precision and relatively cheaply. The data can be elicited from patients far more easily than by using such alternatives as symptom diaries, which may cause severe problems with compliance. The difficulty is that the effects of formaldehyde may not be detectable with this measure because they are likely to occur shortly after exposure and dissipate rapidly, and so they have vanished by the time patients arrive at the clinical setting for testing. Also, relatively large changes in pulmonary function, on the order of 20%, are required to show any effect on patients' function. For a similar reason, the use of death as an endpoint, however important, is unlikely to be sensitive to any subtle changes resulting from low-level exposure. Of course, if formaldehyde is suspected as a potential human carcinogen, the use of death as a measure, specifically respiratory cancer death, is uniquely appropriate.

The important implication of these considerations is that issues of measurement are central to much research in epidemiology. The choice of an appropriate measure is a complex exercise in compromise. Just as investigators should be aware of the issues involved in this choice, critical readers of the literature should closely examine the variables used in a reported investigation to determine whether they are appropriate for the research goals.

TYPES OF VARIABLES

When considering issues of measurement, it is useful to make a distinction among different types of variables. Although there are various ways to describe the different variables, the important distinction is between those variables that are **categorical**, such as dead/alive, diseased/normal, or Protestant/Catholic/Jewish/other, and those that are **continuous**, like diastolic blood pressure, hemoglobin level, height, and many subjective states, such as pain, disability, or mood. Categorical variables can only take on certain discrete values. By contrast, continuous variables can, in theory, assume an infinite number of values.

Within these broad classes there is often a further subdivision. Categorical variables are classified into *nominal* variables, which are named categories like dead/alive, male/female, or white/Oriental/African, and *ordinal* (ordered) categories like Stage I/Stage II/Stage III cancer or much improved/improved/same/worse/much worse. The distinction between the two is that there is no order implied for nominal variables—whites are no higher or lower than Orientals or Africans. In contrast, there is a clear order implied in ordinal variables (e.g., staging in cancer).

Continuous variables are also divided into two classes. With *interval* variables, the distance between points has some quantitative meaning so that the difference between a blood pressure of 95 mm Hg and 105 mm Hg is the same as the difference between 110 mm Hg and 120 mm Hg. For *ratio* variables, the ratio of two quantities has meaning (e.g., the ratio of two temperatures expressed in degrees Kelvin). These latter two concepts are understood better by considering violations of the rule. A rating scale going from "much below average" to "much above average" is not an interval variable because the distance between "much below average" and "below average" has no real meaning—it certainly would not be easy to demonstrate, for example, that it is the same as the difference between "average" and "slightly above average." In a similar vein, the ratio of two temperatures expressed in absolute or Kelvin degrees has some meaning, but degrees on the Celsius scale are not ratio variables—20° C is not twice as hot as 10° C.

The distinction between categorical and continuous variables is important because it influences nearly every way we think about them, as will become evident in the remainder of this section. However, the difference between nominal and ordinal variables is only important in the application of some slightly esoteric statistical tests that work for ordered categories but not for nominal categories. Whether a variable is interval or ratio affects how we can interpret the results (we can talk about *differences* with interval variables, and *ratios* with ratio data), but doesn't affect what type of statistics we can use.

MEASUREMENT WITH CATEGORICAL VARIABLES

We began this section on measurement with the suggestion that much of the confusion surrounding the carcinogenic risk of many environmental hazards is a result of inadequate attention paid to the quantification of risk. In this section, we will develop a number of ways to approach the issue of risk assessment. There are two parts to the question: (1) deciding on the appropriate way to **measure** the health effect and (2) deciding on some way to express the **association** between the supposed cause and the outcome.

For the moment let us define the issue a little more precisely. Without getting into the specifics of risks from radiation, PCBs, dioxin, ethylene dibromide, Agent Orange, cell phones, or hydro lines, it would seem apparent that we are being bombarded with all sorts of chemical, electromagnetic, nuclear, and particulate delights that never assaulted our ancestors. That being the case, one possible result of the overall impact of all these insults to the organism would be an increase in the overall rate of cancer during the past century or so. If these pollutants are indeed devastating to our health, it should be reflected in a gradual increase in cancer rates as time passes.

As we shall see, this *seems* simple enough, but it isn't. First, should we count all cases of cancer or all deaths from cancer? After all, to the extent that our therapies are getting better, we might actually be curing some folks, which would make the death rate drop even though there may be just as many or even more cases around. On the other hand, we're also getting better at detecting cancer with methods like Pap smears and mammography, which weren't available a few years or decades ago. The effect of these might be to inflate the apparent number of cases in recent years, although it would have less impact on deaths because by the time someone dies from it, cancer is fairly obvious.

For convenience and convention, we call the counting of cases the measurement of **frequency** and counting of deaths the measurement of **impact**. We will explore the issue of the overall effect of the environment using both these measures by examining the risks of cancer in the 1930s and the first decade of this century to see if we can detect the effect of a (questionably) deteriorating environment.

Measures of Frequency

Measures of frequency focus on the **occurrence** of disease as opposed to the sequelae of disease (in particular, death). There are a number of ways one can approach the counting of disease. The choice is based on the unpleasant reality that it takes some time to do a study, and while the clock is ticking, new folks are unfortunately developing a disease at the same time that some lucky souls are being cured of it (at least for some diseases) and others are dying of it. All this coming-and-going in and out of the study wreaks havoc with any attempt to count who actually has the disease. To overcome this state of affairs, epidemiologists have worked out a few standard ways of counting bodies, warm or otherwise.

To return to our original problem, let's suppose we wish to count all cases of cancer (of all types) in Canada in 2009. Having agreed on the criteria for diagnosis and carefully set up a sampling frame that is perfectly representative of the population of Canada, or alternatively, having developed a reporting mechanism for all cases in Canada, we now start counting on January 1 and stop on December 31. All the counts come pouring in, and the systems analysts and statisticians are rubbing their hands in glee at all the years of prospective employment ahead. Now the embarrassing questions emerge.

To illustrate the difficulty, let's examine what happened at the cancer reporting center in Plumcoulee, Manitoba. There are a total of 200 people

Table 4-1
Reports of Cancer in Plumcoulee, Manitoba

Patient	Jan	Feb	Mar	Apr	May	Jun	Jul	Aug	Sep	Oct	Nov	Dec
1		▬	▬	▬	X							
2			D	▬	▬	▬	▬	▬	▬	X		
3		▬	▬	▬	▬	▬	▬	▬	▬	▬	▬	▬
4		▬	▬	▬	▬	▬	▬	▬	▬	X		
5						D ▬ C						
6			D	▬	▬	▬	▬	X				
7		▬	C									
8				D	▬	▬	▬	▬	▬	▬	▬	▬
9				D	▬	▬	▬	▬	▬	X		
10											D ▬	
11							D	▬	▬	C		
12		D	▬	X								

D, First diagnosis; ▬, with disease; *C*, cured; *X*, died.

in this farming community, a fact that we'll need to know later. The reports to the center are shown in Table 4-1.

It is obvious from the table that we can get wildly different estimates of the amount of cancer in Plumcoulee depending on how we choose to do the counting. If we just look at the number of cases around at any point in time, we find 4 in January, 3 in December, and 8 in July. If we count the total number of folks who were reported this year, the answer is 12. If we count the number of new cases in 1987, it's 8. Finally, there were 6 deaths from cancer in that year.

There are, however, some standard ways to report the data, as we'll discuss in this section.

Incidence

Incidence is defined as follows:

$$\text{Incidence} = \frac{\text{Number of new cases in a fixed time period}}{\text{Number of people at risk}}$$

Usually the period of study is chosen to be 1 year, in which case we speak of the **annual incidence**. In Plumcoulee (Table 4-1) there were eight new cases of cancer in 2009. If we had decided to focus on the 3-month incidence, there were three new cases from January to March.

The denominator, or number of people at risk, is not quite 200 people because patients 1, 3, 4, and 7 already had cancer and thus could not be counted as "at risk"; this reduces the denominator to 196. Thus the annual incidence is as follows:

$$\text{Annual Incidence} = \frac{8}{196} = 0.0408 \text{ cases a year}$$

Usually the incidence of disease is much lower than in this example, and the correction for preexisting cases is unnecessary. Further, to make things more readable, incidence is often cited as cases per 1000 (in this example, 40.8 cases per 1000 a year) or even as cases per million a year for rare disorders.

Prevalence

If we are planning screening programs, disease incidence is of immediate interest. However, if we are concerned with the provision of services for people with the disease, such as palliative care, our immediate concern is "How many people actually have the disease at any point in time?" This quantity is called the **prevalence**, which is defined as follows:

$$\text{Prevalence} = \frac{\text{Number of people with the disease}}{\text{Number of people at risk}}$$

In contrast to incidence, prevalence is determined at a single point in time. Still considering the data from Table 4-1, perhaps the most rational point in time to choose is the middle of 2009, or July 1. Looking at the table, we find that patients 2, 3, 4, 6, 8, and 9 had cancer at this time. Patient 5 was cured sometime in July, and should be counted on July 1, whereas patient 11 was diagnosed in July and would likely not enter the count. This leaves a total of seven cases in the numerator.

Again the denominator is not quite 200. By July 1, patients 1 and 12 were deceased, so the denominator is only 198. Finally, the prevalence is as follows:

$$\text{Prevalence} = \frac{7}{198} = 0.0354 = 35.4 \text{ per } 1000$$

Period Prevalence

A close analogy to the incidence is the **period prevalence**, which is based on the number of people with the disease during a defined period of time (usually 1 year). The formal definition is as follows:

$$\text{Prevalence} = \frac{\text{Number of people with the disease during the time period}}{\text{Number of people at risk during the time period}}$$

The calculation of annual prevalence in our example from Table 4-1 is straightforward. There are 12 people identified as having cancer in that year and 200 at risk, so the period prevalence is simply 12/200 = 0.06 = 60 per 1000. If we were to calculate the quarterly prevalence for the first quarter of the year, we would include only patients 1, 2, 3, 4, 6, 7, and 12; the period prevalence for 3 months is therefore 7/200 = 0.035 = 35 per 1000.

Relation Between Prevalence and Incidence

The previous definitions were slightly different in dimensions. Incidence is based on a fixed time period and is quoted per month or year. However, prevalence is calculated at a single point in time. It happens that the two quantities have the following interesting relationship, which involves the average duration of disease:

$$\text{Prevalence} = \text{Incidence} \times \text{Duration}$$

It's not easy to demonstrate the relationship mathematically, but it is easy to show that it is reasonable. Think of a chronic but relatively non-lethal disease like rheumatoid arthritis (RA). Once an individual acquires the disease, he or she carries it until death, so the duration is calculated by subtracting the average age at onset from the expected life span. Thus each new case of RA is added to the pool of prevalent cases, and although relatively few cases may be added each year, there are a large number of prevalent cases around. So the prevalence of RA is much greater than annual incidence.

By contrast, the ordinary cold has a duration of a few days at most, and kids can often get more than one a year. In this situation the annual incidence might approach, or even exceed, 1000 per 1000. Yet unless there's an epidemic around, relatively few people have a cold at any time, so the prevalence of colds is not nearly as high as the incidence—perhaps 50 per 1000. Because the duration is short, the prevalence is much lower than the annual incidence.

The relationship may seem to be of only arcane interest. However, it is often easier to obtain published data on disease prevalence than on incidence; yet if you want to do an intervention or prevention study, it is usually of greater interest to know how many new cases you are likely to get. Through the use of this formula and a reasoned guess at the duration of the disease, you can arrive at a plausible estimate of the number of new cases.

Case Fatality Rate

While we're examining the fate of the Plumcoulee patients from Table 4-1, we might as well introduce a term that links disease *frequency*, or the likelihood of developing the disease, to disease *impact*, or the likelihood of dying from the disease.

First of all we note that a total of six persons from Plumcoulee died of cancer during the study. It is natural to express this quantity in a similar manner to our measures of disease occurrence to form a quantity called the **mortality rate**, which is defined as follows:

$$\text{Mortality Rate} = \frac{\text{Number of deaths from disease in a time period}}{\text{Number of people at risk}}$$

Studying the data from Plumcoulee, we see that six people (patients 1, 2, 4, 6, 9, and 12) died of cancer in 2009. There were 200 people at risk so the **annual mortality rate** was 6/200 = 0.03, or 30 per 1000.

As we shall see in the discussion on measures of impact, this approach is a fairly crude basis for comparison. However, there is another relationship evident from the display. When relating frequency to impact we might wish to study the likelihood that a disease may be fatal. This quantity is called the **case fatality rate** and is defined as follows:

$$\text{Case Fatality Rate} = \frac{\text{Number of deaths from disease in a time period}}{\text{Number of people with the disease}}$$

In the present example, there were 12 people with cancer in Plumcoulee in 2009 and 6 deaths; the case fatality rate is therefore 6/12 = 50% a year.

Measures of Impact

We began this discussion with the idea that one broad way to determine whether all the industrial pollutants have affected human health was to examine the rates of cancer during several decades to see if any increasing trend was evident. We briefly discussed the advantages and disadvantages of looking at disease frequency (cases of cancer) and disease impact (deaths from cancer).

The impact of disease need not focus entirely on death. For a chronic disease like arthritis, disease impact would more appropriately be calculated using measures of activities of daily living, function, or quality of life. However, for the example we have been pursuing, we will focus on mortality. The measurement of mortality has one major advantage over the measurement of frequency, namely that relatively complete archival sources are available and have been for several decades (or for several centuries in Great Britain). Instead of setting up a reporting system such as was proposed for Plumcoulee and allowing it to run for a few decades while we epidemiologists cool our collective heels, we can conduct a retrospective impact study.

In this discussion we use actual data, based on Canadian statistics for 1933 and 1973, to examine our research hypothesis that the increased level of chemical, radiologic, and particulate pollution in Canada in the intervening 40 years has led to an increase in the observed rate of death from cancer.

Mortality Rate

To test this hypothesis, let's turn to our desk copy of Canadian statistics. We look up the appropriate sections and compile the data (Table 4-2). To make the comparison easier, it makes sense to work out the number of deaths per 1000 population. This is called the annual mortality rate, which is defined as follows:

$$\text{Annual Mortality Rate} = \frac{\text{Number of deaths in a year}}{\text{Total population}}$$

For 1933 the annual mortality rate is 11,056 per 10,500,000, or 1.05 per 1000. For 1973 the annual mortality rate is 44,877 per 21,400,000, or 2.10 per 1000. From these data it would appear that the rate of cancer has nearly doubled in 40 years. We may conclude that perhaps there is evidence of a significant health effect of pollutants. Nevertheless, there are a number of steps we can take to refine the comparison.

Proportional Mortality Rate

We were in a fortunate position when we calculated the mortality rate to have a good estimate of the denominator, or the population at risk. Federal census takers in the Western world go to great pains and expense to determine how many people there are in the country in given years (perhaps so they can ensure complete tax returns to pay for the census). However, in many situations where research is conducted on subpopulations (e.g., workers exposed to welding fumes or residents near a landfill site), it would be difficult or impossible to determine on the basis of existing records how many people were in the denominator in a given year.

Table 4-2
Canadian Cancer Statistics

	1933	1973
Total population	10,500,000	21,400,000
Deaths from cancer	11,056	44,877

From National Cancer Institute of Canada: Canadian cancer statistics, Toronto, 1995, NCIC.

On the other hand, it is much easier to determine the causes of death of all the people in a population who died because death certificates are a legal necessity. We can reason that if pollutants are causing more cancer in 1973 than they did in 1933, proportionately more deaths should be caused by cancer than by other causes in 1973 than in 1933. This approach is called the **proportional mortality rate (PMR)**. It requires no knowledge of the people at risk, only mortality data. The PMR is defined as follows:

$$PMR = \frac{\text{Number of deaths from a particular cause}}{\text{Total number of deaths}}$$

It turns out that in 1933 there were a total of 122,850 deaths recorded in Canada. In 1973, 236,200 deaths were recorded. The resultant PMRs are shown in Table 4-3.

It appears that the same trend to higher mortality rates in 1973 is present in these data. Of course one alternative explanation is that proportionately more people were dying of cancer in 1973 simply because fewer people were dying from everything else. This makes some sense because tuberculosis, diphtheria, and other serious infectious diseases were present in 1933 but absent in 1973. Centainly there is some evidence that this may be occurring; men born in 1933 had a life expectancy of 41.1 years, whereas men born in 1973 had a life expectancy of 68.2 years.

This example also nicely illustrates the strengths and weaknesses of the PMR method. Its strength is that it can be applied in situations in which only minimal data are available; its weakness is that a high PMR is always open to two interpretations: (1) more deaths from the cause of interest or (2) fewer deaths from everything else.

Age-Specific Mortality

In general, cancer is a disease of old age. Although a few young persons die of cancer, in most circumstances there is a period of a few decades between exposure to some cancer-causing agent and the onset of the disease.

Table 4-3
Proportional Mortality Rates for Cancer

Total deaths	122,850	236,200
Deaths from cancer	11,056	44,877
Proportional mortality rate	9.0%	19.0%

From National Cancer Institute of Canada: Canadian cancer statistics, Toronto, 1995, NCIC.

This must be kept in mind when contrasting 1933 with 1973; not only might more people have died from other causes in 1933, as we mentioned previously, but also more people might have died young from other causes and not lived long enough to develop cancer.

To determine if this reasoning results in an alternative explanation for the higher observed cancer mortality in 1973, we could look only at the death rate from cancer in older people (e.g., older than 75 years of age). We could then calculate the cancer mortality rate in this age segment. The result is called the **age-specific mortality rate**, which is defined as follows:

$$\text{Age-Specific Mortality Rate} = \frac{\text{Number of deaths in a particular age range}}{\text{Total number of deaths in a particular age range}}$$

Let's work this example through. In 1933 there were 5126 Canadians older than 75; in this group there were 110 cancer deaths. Therefore the age-specific mortality rate is 110/5126 = 21.5 per 1000. Similar data from 1973 indicate that there were 915 cancer deaths among the 35,295 Canadians older than age 75, which results in an age-specific mortality rate of 915/35,295 = 25.9 per 1000.

These rates are indeed a little closer than the overall mortality rates we looked at earlier, thereby suggesting that a partial explanation for the differences is simply that people were dying of other causes in 1933 and were not living long enough to develop cancer. However, it is unfortunate that in order to make this comparison it was necessary to ignore most of the data.

Standardized Mortality Rate

The discussion on age-specific mortality rate suggested that if we restricted our view to those individuals who survived long enough to be at risk of developing cancer, there was a smaller difference in cancer rates between 1933 and 1973 than was evident when we simply looked at overall mortality. The difference between the two sets of data reflects (1) the influence of age on mortality rates from a specific disease and (2) differences in the age distributions between the Canadian population in 1933 and 1973.

Most diseases show a strong relationship with age. Risk from chronic diseases like heart disease and cancer increases with age, whereas infectious diseases are more common in the young. Even pedestrian mortality shows a strong bimodal distribution with age and strikes the very young, who lack awareness of the dangers of traffic, and the very old, who can no longer see and hear danger as well as before (or run as fast!).

Because of the strong influence of age on disease mortality rates, any comparison between two different populations is considerably strengthened by correcting for the differences in age distribution. This approach is called the **standardized mortality rate** (**SMR**) and builds on the age-specific mortality rate. Having broken down the deaths in the population of interest by age and created age-specific mortality rates, we then use them with the distribution of age in a reference or standard population to create an overall projected mortality rate. These are the four basis steps in the process:

1. Calculate the age-specific mortality rate for each age range in the population of interest.
2. Multiply this rate by the number of people in the age range in the standard population. This result then determines the number of individuals in the standard population who would die from the disease.
3. Add up the total number of projected deaths across all age levels of the standard population.
4. Finally, convert this sum to a mortality rate by dividing by the total numbers in the standard population.

For example, to compare the cancer mortality in 1933 and 1973, we will project them both onto a reference population distribution (in this case the population distribution of Canada in 1970, but any year could have been chosen). The method is illustrated in Table 4-4.

After this lengthy process we then can determine that the standardized mortality rate for cancer deaths in 1933 is 2510 per 1 million, or 2.51 per 1000. Similar calculations can be performed for cancer deaths

Table 4-4
Calculations for Standardized Mortality Rate

1 Age Range	2 1933 Pop	3 Cancer Deaths	4 Age-Specific Mortality (Col. 3 ÷ Col. 2)	5 1970 Pop	6 Standard Deaths (Col. 4 × Col. 5)
0–4	49,113	2	0.000041	84,416	3.44
5–9	42,014	4	0.000095	98,204	9.35
•					
•					
•					
75–79	2,891	41	0.014182	18,871	267.6
80–84	1,403	40	0.028510	11,241	320.5
>84	832	29	0.034856	7,435	259.2
Total				1,000,000	2,510

From National Cancer Institute of Canada: Canadian cancer statistics, Toronto, 1995, NCIC.

in 1973 and from all other causes in both 1933 and 1973 always using the 1970 population as the standard. These calculations are shown in Table 4-5.

Some of our suspicions are therefore correct. People indeed died at a much faster rate from other causes in 1933 than in 1973—15.12 per 1000 versus 8.91 per 1000, respectively. There nevertheless appears to be an excess cancer risk persisting in 1973 of approximately 20% (3.10 versus 2.51 per 1000). However, this is considerably less than the doubled risk originally calculated using the unstandardized mortality rates.

In summary, the SMR is about the best estimate of the mortality arising from a particular cause and is virtually a prerequisite for any comparison across different populations. Proportional mortality rates are a weak alternative, useful only in situations in which there are no denominator data available.

It should be kept in mind that the application of SMRs corrects for the confounding effect of age, and possibly of sex differences, but that's all. To conclude that *any* observed difference results from a particular cause requires the elimination of all other possible causes. The point is nicely illustrated by a final run at the 1933–1973 comparison.

The difficulty arises from the use of a historical control, as described in Chapter 3. To conclude that the observed difference between 1933 and 1973 is caused by industrial pollution requires that we eliminate from suspicion all the other differences between 1933 and 1973. One difference in particular is staring us in the face—cigarette smoking. Smoking per capita has increased steadily from the turn of the century until recent times, and cigarettes are a known and strong causal factor in lung cancer. These facts suggest that we may further understand the cause of the increase of cancer deaths from 1933 to 1973 by separating respiratory cancer from cancers of all other sites (because the latter are only weakly related to smoking). If we do this and calculate SMRs for respiratory cancer and other sites, all the differences between 1973 and 1933 can be accounted for by a sevenfold difference in respiratory cancer rates (Table 4-6). This of course doesn't prove that smoking, rather than pollution, is the cause of the increase. However, it does suggest that there is no general impact of air, water, and foodborne chemicals on human health reflected in cancer rates.

Table 4-5
Standardized Mortality Rates per 1000

	1933	1973
Cancer	2.51	3.10
All other causes	15.12	8.91

Table 4-6
Respiratory Cancers versus Cancers from All Other Sites*

	1933	1973
Respiratory	0.09	0.69
Other sites	2.42	2.41
Total	2.51	3.10

*Standardized mortality rates per 1000

Measures of Association with Categorical Variables

We began this discussion with the assertion that much of our fear about cancer and the environment was a result of inadequate quantification of the additional risk. To this point, we have dwelt on measurement issues and sought means to measure the health effects in an unbiased manner. We now wish to explore methods to measure the *strength of association* between two variables.

We have already used some rough-and-ready measures of association. We found in the last section that there was a sevenfold higher risk of respiratory cancer in 1973 than in 1933. We could restate the data in two other ways: (1) the risk of respiratory cancer increased from 0.09 per 1000 to 0.69 per 1000 or (2) there was a risk of cancer of 0.60 per 1000 attributed to the different circumstances in 1973 and 1933. In the next few examples, we will formalize these concepts.

Let's begin with a new example that is related to therapeutic benefit. The issue is the relationship between cholesterol and heart disease. For a long time a strong association between serum cholesterol and heart disease has been known; however, the implications of this finding were not clear. Did a high level of cholesterol "cause" heart disease or was it simply a marker of a certain genetic predisposition? The key issue has been whether it could be demonstrated that lowering cholesterol levels by diet or drugs would reduce the rate of heart disease.

This was finally demonstrated in 1985 by the Coronary Primary Prevention Trial (CPPT), a randomized trial that was conducted at a number of clinics in North America. The researchers began by screening nearly half a million men to find a group of 3900 who had high serum cholesterol levels (above 256 mg dL) but as yet no evidence of disease. The men also had to comply with a fierce regimen. The drug, called cholestyramine, was foul-smelling, foul-tasting, and gut-wrenching, and had to be taken in water six times a day. The researchers eventually found their bunch of docile souls who would go along with the treatment. They were randomized into two groups (the placebo was concocted to taste just as bad) and followed for 7 to 10 years. After the dust settled there were 30 cardiac deaths in the drug group and 38 in the control group, figures that were statistically significant. There was no overall difference in death rates, but this won't concern us.

Not surprisingly, cholestyramine was not a big hit. But it took several more generations of lipid-lowering drugs and several more hundreds of millions of research dollars before a practical one hit the market. These are the famous "statins," which are now so mainstream that the day may come when they're in the water supply. About the most convincing evidence that they're good for you (and cholesterol is bad for you) came from a large study done in the west of Scotland, the WOSCOP trial, reported in 1995.

They began with a seriously at-risk population—fish-and-chips-loving Scots—and then upped the odds of a heart attack still more by finding a group of middle-aged men (that helps) with elevated total cholesterol (average 7 mmol/l). They were followed for five years, and then they counted bodies. Looking at definite and suspected cardiac deaths (for the moment), there were 61 coronary heart deaths in the placebo group and 41 in the statin group ($p = 0.042$, whew, just made it). If you go to just definite coronary deaths, it's 52 to 38, $p = 0.13$. If you go the other direction, to overall mortality, it's 135 to 106, $p = 0.051$ (darn, just missed it). Unlike the cholestyramine trial, then, (a) folks were just popping a pill with few side effects, not swallowing plastic crud, and (b) there was some effect on overall mortality. It's still interesting to note that this was the best of the trials, and led to millions of consumers consuming statins—even those without high cholesterol or other risk factors.

But this is not the time for philosophy. Let's see how we can summarize these numbers into measures of overall effectiveness. The ways in which these data might be displayed are discussed next.

Relative Risk

The data from the WOSCOP study appear in Table 4-7. The **relative risk** (**RR**), as the name implies, is a measure of the likelihood of occurrence of the target event (death or disease) in those exposed and not exposed to the agent of interest. It is defined as follows:

$$RR = \frac{\text{Mortality rate } \left(\text{or incidence}\right) \text{ in exposed group}}{\text{Mortality rate } \left(\text{or incidence}\right) \text{ in unexposed group}}$$

Coronary mortality rates in the two groups are 61 out of 3293 in the unexposed (placebo) group, and 41 of 3302 in the statin group. Therefore the relative risk for provistatin is $41/3302 \div 61/3293$ or 0.67. To put it another way, the risk of cardiac death in the treated group was $1.00 - 0.76$ or 33% lower than in the placebo group, so the **risk reduction** was 33%.

The data can be presented in another way. We could turn the question around and ask what the RR of cardiac death resulting from the absence of a drug is. This RR is the inverse of the previous calculation: $61/3293 \div 41/3302 = 1.49$. Just to write this out more formally, the RR is as follows:

$$RR = \frac{\dfrac{A}{A+B}}{\dfrac{C}{C+D}} = \frac{A(C+D)}{C(A+B)}$$

Despite the fact that researchers and clinicians love the RR, and prefer it over other indices, such as the relative odds or odds ratio (discussed in a bit), it has a serious, and some would say fatal, limitation. Let's use the same data in Table 4-7, but express the outcome in terms of survival, rather than deaths. We would hope that the answer is simply the reciprocal of 0.670 (which is 1.493), but it's not; it is 1.006. Thus, it makes a big difference whether we frame the answer in terms of risk of dying or risk of surviving, which is not at all reassuring.

Etiologic Fraction

Closely related to the notion of risk reduction is a concept called the **etiologic fraction (EF)**. When considering a risk factor for a disease, in this case untreated high cholesterol levels, we are interested in what fraction of the cases of cardiac death has untreated high cholesterol levels as its etiology. Because there were 61 deaths in this group when high cholesterol levels were present and 41 deaths when this risk factor was absent (assuming the drug worked for all people), we could define the proportion of cardiac deaths, or the EF, as follows:

$$EF = \frac{\text{Mortality in exposed group} - \text{Mortality in unexposed group}}{\text{Mortality in exposed group}}$$

Table 4-7
Data from the WOSCOP Study

	Cardiac Deaths	Alive	
Provistatin	41 (A)	3261 (B)	3302
Placebo	61 (C)	3232 (D)	3293

From Muntoni S: Cholesterol-lowering drugs for primary prevention: the WOSCOP Study. *Pharmacol* Res 35: 169–170, 1997.

For the WOSCOP trial (Table 4-7), the etiological fraction is (61 − 41) / 61 = 33%. This is the same number as, although a different concept than, the risk reduction we calculated earlier.

Attributable Risk

The RR gives some indication of the increased risk (in the case of a risk factor) or benefit (in the case of a therapy) in relative terms. However, we would often like to examine the actual increase or reduction in incidence or mortality attributed to the cause. This is called the **attributable risk (AR)** and is defined as follows:

$$AR = \begin{array}{c} \text{Mortality rate (or incidence)} \\ \text{in exposed group} \end{array} - \begin{array}{c} \text{Mortality rate (or incidence)} \\ \text{in unexposed group} \end{array}$$

In the previous example (Table 4-7), the attributable risk of cardiac death (attributable to untreated high cholesterol) is 61/3293 − 41/3302 = 6.1 per 1000.

The example nicely illustrates the important differences between the two concepts of RR and AR. The WOSCOP trial began with a highly selected cohort of people with high cholesterol levels, followed them for a long time (five years), and indeed demonstrated a statistically significant risk reduction of 33%. However, this amounted to a reduction in risk of cardiac death of only 6 per 1000, compared with a total rate of death in both groups of approximately 31 per 1000.

Number Needed to Treat

When we're dealing with the effects of some form of therapy, the AR (which is also called the **absolute risk reduction [ARR]**) is good for telling us how much of the improvement is due to the intervention, as opposed to that other powerful treatment, the natural healing process of the body (for which we cannot bill). However, it's difficult to translate the ARR into a treatment plan; *is it worth giving a statin for an ARR of 0.006?*

A neat way to make the number more meaningful was proposed by Laupacis and his group and consists simply of taking the inverse of the ARR. This then becomes the **number needed to treat (NNT)**. So an ARR of 0.006 becomes an NNT of 1.0 / 0.006 = 167, which means that we would have to treat 167 patients with a statin for five years in order to save one life. To see how this works, the ARR can be interpreted that we have to treat one person to save 0.006 lives, or 1000 persons to save (1000 × 0.006) = 6 lives. So we must treat 1000/6 = 167, to save one life. Now the clinician has to decide whether the benefit of saving the life of one patient is counterbalanced by the risk of side effects (and cost) to the 166 people who will survive anyway without the drug.

Relative Odds

The concepts of association we have discussed so far work well for most situations in which we wish to examine the effect of a particular risk factor on the subsequent occurrence of disease. However, there is one study design, the case-control study (see Chapter 3), in which things don't quite fit. Case-control studies are used in situations in which the likelihood of developing disease is low or there is a long latency before the onset of disease. Typically, both these conditions apply to the investigation of risk factors in cancer. In these circumstances, we assemble a group of people with the disease (cases) and an appropriate set of people without disease (controls), usually of the same size, and we examine the exposure of the two groups to the risk factor of interest.

As one example, continuing our cancer theme, Table 4-8 was derived from one of the original studies linking lung cancer to smoking. The fact that the rate of lung cancer overall is so high is a sure clue that we are dealing with a case-control study because if these data were based on a cohort study that assembled persons who did and didn't smoke, we would arrive at the alarming conclusion that the overall rate of lung cancer was approximately 34%. However, if we continue along the lines we had done previously, we could calculate a risk of cancer in the exposed group of 659/684, or 96%, and in the unexposed group of 984/1332, or 74%. The RR of lung cancer is then, using the previous methods, 0.96/0.74 = 1.30. Although the final result seems plausible, the intermediate steps are insane because of the nature of the design. In fact, lung cancer is much rarer than we have made it out to be; the controls without cancer are sampled from a much larger population of healthy folks than are the cases.

Table 4-8
Lung Cancer and Smoking

	Cases	Controls	Total
Smoker	659	984	1643
	A	B	
	C	D	
Nonsmoker	25	348	373
Total	684	1332	2016

From Wynder EL, Graham EA: Tobacco smoking as a possible etiologic factor in bronchogenic carcinoma: a study of 684 proved cases, JAMA 143:329–336, 1950.

Although we cannot calculate from these data an actual risk of getting lung cancer, we can frame things in a different way. We begin with the cases and play a gambling game, asking the odds that this person was exposed to the suspected carcinogen. When a gambler says that the odds of a candidate's being elected are 1:4, he or she is saying that the probability of the person being elected is one-quarter that of not being elected, and because these probabilities add to one, a little mental arithmetic shows that the probability that this candidate will be elected is 20%. Similarly, the odds that an individual with lung cancer was exposed to tobacco are A/C = 659/25 = 26.4; and the odds that an individual in the control group was exposed is B/D = 984/348 = 2.83. The **relative odds (RO)** of lung cancer from tobacco exposure are then as follows:

$$RO = \frac{\text{Odds of exposure for cases}}{\text{Odds of exposure for controls}} = \frac{A/C}{B/D}$$
$$= 26.4 / 2.83$$
$$= 9.33$$

The more common way to write the equation for the RO is as follows:

$$RO = \frac{AD}{BC}$$

The RO, which is also called the **odds ratio (OR)** is usually higher than the RR. Whether this is a bad or a good thing depends on which index you regard as "truth." As we said, most clinicians opt for the RR, but some have argued in favor of the RO. One major reason is that it doesn't suffer from the shortcoming we mentioned for the RR, that it is not symmetrical with respect to using the good outcome or the bad outcome as the end-point. That is, if we recalculate the RO in Table 4-8 using the controls in the numerator rather than the cases, we get an answer of 0.107, which is simply the reciprocal of 9.33. So the RO meets the symmetry criterion, which the RR does not. However, when the prevalence of the disorder we're looking at is fairly low, the two are pretty close to one another. The reason is that, under these circumstances, A + B is close to B, and C + D is close to D (because cells A and C record the prevalence). Therefore the formulae for the RR and the RO (or OR) come out the same.

Diagnostic Tests

The twentieth century has seen dramatic changes in disease patterns in the Western world. Since the advent of effective antibiotics, vaccines, and, perhaps most important, adequate nutrition and sanitation, most people in industrialized countries can look forward to a full life. Our present preoccupation is with chronic, lifestyle-related diseases for which there are unlikely to be any "magic bullets" in the foreseeable future.

One result of these changes is that epidemiologists have moved away from their historical roots in the study of epidemics to such diverse activities as the study of occupational risks or trials of therapeutic agents in order to maintain employment. (One result of this shift in employment patterns is that books such as this one are now required to tell health professionals what epidemiologists do.)

However, thanks to a new infectious disease, acquired immunodeficiency syndrome (AIDS), that has all the devastating characteristics of the traditional scourges of mankind, like cholera and the black plague, epidemiologists find themselves the center of attention at cocktail parties. We need not devote any space in this section to describing the natural history, prevalence, modes of transmission, or risk factors of AIDS—these are taught to elementary school students. However, we will use this disease as an instructive example of a measurement problem, the application of diagnostic tests.

There are now two high-risk populations for AIDS—homosexuals because of sexual contact and street drug users because of the sharing of contaminated needles. Before the advent of adequate screening tests, there was a third high-risk segment—people requiring blood transfusions for any reason. In particular, a significant number of hemophiliacs acquired AIDS as a result of their exposure to large numbers of transfusions. However, since 1985 all blood products are routinely screened for positive human immunodeficiency virus (HIV+) antibodies using the enzyme-linked immunosorbent assay (ELISA) test.

As screening tests go, ELISA is a good one indeed. This is fortunate because the consequences of the test are severe. If an individual has HIV antibodies, there is a 100% chance of eventually developing the disease, and AIDS has nearly a 100% mortality. The consequences of a false positive are also severe. If we tell someone he or she has antibodies when this isn't the case, we are causing massive anxiety and lifestyle changes. Conversely, if we miss blood products containing antibodies, the chance of infecting someone is high.

Let us examine the performance of this test in two populations: (1) in a homosexual population in which the prevalence of HIV antibodies is approximately 50% and (2) in routine screening of blood donations in which the prevalence of antibodies is approximately 0.2%.

True Positive, False Positive, True Negative, and False Negative Rates

Let us imagine that the ELISA test is being used as a screening test for a high-risk population (e.g., homosexuals in New York City). Actual figures for this group indicate that the prevalence of the HIV antibody is approximately 50%.

To examine the test performance, we could screen a group of individuals and compare the test result with their true status. Truth isn't easy to come by, but in this case there is a more expensive but virtually perfect test called the Western blot test. We could take samples from the group and perform both tests on the samples. If we were to screen 1000 individuals with the test and compare the test result with the "gold standard," the results would be similar to those found in Table 4-9.

The characteristics of tests are usually described in terms of the letters (A, B, C, D) in the four cells of the table. One way of describing the test's performance is as follows:

$$\textbf{True Positive Rate} = \frac{\text{People with positive test and disease}}{\text{All people with disease}}$$
$$= A/(A + C) = 498/508$$
$$= 98.03 \text{ percent}$$

$$\textbf{False Negative Rate} = \frac{\text{People with negative test and disease}}{\text{All people with disease}}$$
$$= C/(A + C) = 10/508$$
$$= 1.97 \text{ percent}$$

Table 4-9
Results of ELISA versus Western Blot Text in Screening of 1000 Homosexuals from New York City

| | Gold Standard (Western Blot) | | |
	Antibodies	No Antibodies	Total
Positive	498 (A)	4 (B)	502
Negative	10 (C)	48 (D)	498
Total	508	492	1000

$$\textbf{True Negative Rate} = \frac{\text{People with negative test and no disease}}{\text{All people without disease}}$$

$$= D/(B + D) = 488/492$$
$$= 99.19 \text{ percent}$$

$$\textbf{False Positive Rate} = \frac{\text{People with positive test and no disease}}{\text{All people without disease}}$$

$$= B/(B + D) = 4/492$$
$$= 0.81 \text{ percent}$$

Sensitivity and Specificity

Another way of describing the test's characteristics has its origins in the biochemistry laboratory. We speak of **sensitivity**—how sensitive the test is at detecting disease—and **specificity**—how good the test is at rejecting samples that are not diseased. Let's use the data from Table 4-9.

The sensitivity is a measure of the test's ability to detect people with the disease and is measured as follows:

$$\text{Sensitivity} = \frac{\text{Number with disease who have a positive test}}{\text{Number with disease}}$$
$$= A/(A + C) = 498/508$$
$$= 98.03 \text{ percent}$$

Conversely, the specificity measures the ability of the test to correctly identify people who do not have the disease and is measured as follows:

$$\text{Specificity} = \frac{\text{Number without disease who have a negative test}}{\text{Number without disease}}$$
$$= D/(B + D) = 488/492$$
$$= 99.19 \text{ percent}$$

As you can see, sensitivity is the same as true positive rate, and specificity is the same as true negative rate.

Positive and Negative Predictive Values

The descriptions thus far give some picture of the characteristics of the test. However, the denominator for both sensitivity and specificity assumes some knowledge of the true state of affairs because it is based on people who do or don't have the disease. Clinicians rarely have the luxury of a "gold standard"; if they did, they wouldn't be doing the test. Putting it another way, assume you are about to advise someone who has just received a positive ELISA. Do you tell the individual that he or she has HIV antibodies? What is the chance that someone with a positive ELISA does not have antibodies? These probabilities are embodied in the concepts of **positive predictive value** and **negative predictive value**, in which the denominators are based on people with positive and negative tests. Again using the data from Table 4-9, these values are measured as follows:

$$\text{Positive Predictive Value} = \frac{\text{People with positive test and disease}}{\text{All people with positive test}}$$
$$= A/(A + B)$$
$$= 498/502$$
$$= 99.20 \text{ percent}$$
$$\text{Negative Predictive Value} = \frac{\text{People with negative test and no disease}}{\text{All people with negative test}}$$
$$= D/(C + D)$$
$$= 488/498$$
$$= 97.99 \text{ percent}$$

Relationship Between Prevalence and Predictive Value

The data we have presented so far give a fairly encouraging picture of the ELISA test. If someone has a positive test, we can be 99.2% certain that person really has HIV antibodies. However, the calculations were based on a situation where the prevalence of antibodies was high (approximately 50%). In different circumstances the picture may not be as rosy. For example, experience in screening blood donations has shown that the prevalence of AIDS antibodies is actually closer to 0.2%. As pointed out more than 5 decades ago, this change in prevalence may drastically affect the usefulness of the test.

Working out a new contingency table (as in Table 4-9), we now have a prevalence of 0.2%; two people out of the 1000 will have antibodies, and 998 will not. Because the prevalence is so low, imagine screening 1,000,000 units of blood, of which approximately 2000 will have antibodies (whether we use 1000 samples or 1,000,000 does not affect the results at all, it just eliminates decimal points during the calculations). Because the test has a sensitivity of 98.0%, $0.98 \times 2000 = 1960$ persons will test positive with ELISA (cell A) and 40 will test negative (cell C). Now there will be $1,000,000 - 2000$, or 998,000 normal units of blood. We know from our previous data that the specificity of the test is 99.2%; there will be a total of $0.992 \times 998,000 = 990,016$ normal units that test negative (cell D). Conversely, there will be $998,000 - 990,016 = 7984$ normal units of blood that have positive ELISA tests (cell B). The new data appear in Table 4-10.

If we now recalculate the predictive values, they look like the following:

| Positive Predictive Value | = | 1960/9944 | = | 19.7% |
| Negative Predictive Value | = | 990,016/990,056 | = | 99.99% |

The picture is now different than in the first situation. If a person has a negative test, there is virtual certainty that he or she truly is HIV negative. However, a positive test is nearly uninterpretable because more than 80% of the positive test results come from people who don't have antibodies!

In actual practice any blood that tests positive is sent for a repeat ELISA and a Western blot test. If ELISA remains positive and the Western blot is negative, the blood is discarded but the donor is not told. If they are both positive, the donor is informed and contacts are traced.

Thus, in general, the prevalence of disease has a profound effect on the usefulness of a test. If the prevalence is low, the positive predictive value of the test is low and the negative predictive value high. Conversely, if the prevalence of disease is high, the negative predictive value is low but the positive predictive value is high.

A prime example of a beautiful test being wrecked on the shoals of low prevalence rates is one that detects levels of the protein CA 125 in women with ovarian cancer. It has a sensitivity of 100% and a specificity over 95%. However, because the prevalence of ovarian cancer in women over 35 years of age is less than 1 in 2,500, the positive predictive value is under 1%—over 99% of the women "diagnosed" by the test would be perfectly normal.

Incremental Validity

In Table 4-10, the Negative Predictive Value looks pretty impressive; the ELISA test is picking up 99.99% of people who don't have antibodies. But

Table 4-10
Prevalence of HIV Antibodies per 1,000,000 Units of Blood

| | | Gold Standard (Western Blot) | | |
		Antibodies	No Antibodies	Total
ELISA	Positive	1960 (A)	7984 (B)	9944
	Negative	40 (C)	990 016 (D)	990,056
	Total	2000	998,000	1,000,000

wait a second. Let's say we didn't have ELISA available to us; we just close our eyes and say "No Antibodies" for every sample that crosses our desk. Much to the amazement of our peers who haven't read this book, we would be correct 99.80% of the time, because that's the proportion of antibody-free samples. Now that figure of 99.99% doesn't look quite as impressive. What we need is some index that tells us how much the test improves our predictive power over and above the base rate. In fact, there are two such sets of indices.

The **incremental positive (negative) predictive values** are:

Incremental Positive Predictive Value = Positive Predictive Value − Prevalence

Incremental Negative Predictive Value = Negative Predictive Value − (1 − Prevalence)

In our example, the prevalence of antibodies is 0.002, so the Incremental Negative Predictive Value is:

Incremental Negative Predictive Value = 0.9999 − (1 − 0.002) = 0.0019

and we would use the formula for the incremental positive predictive value in high-prevalence situations, when we are interested in the improvement of the positive predictive value.

One problem with these numbers is that it's hard to put a meaning to them. So, Kraemer introduced a variant called the **quality predictive value**:

$$\text{Quality Positive Predictive Value} = \frac{\text{Positive Predictive Value} - \text{Prevalence}}{1 - \text{Prevalence}}$$

$$\text{Quality Negative Predictive Value} = \frac{\text{Negative Predictive Value} - (1 - \text{Prevalence})}{1 - (1 - \text{Prevalence})}$$

Running the same numbers through the formula, we get:

$$\text{Quality Negative Predictive Value} = \frac{.9999 - .9980}{1 - .9980} = 0.95$$

We get a value of 0 when the test tells us nothing over and above the prevalence, and a value of 1.0 when there are no diagnostic errors. In this case, there's a 95% increase in diagnostic value by using ELISA, which ain't bad at all. Not all (or even very many) tests look this good. What we have to balance is the cost of the test against the added improvement in our detection ability.

Bayes's Theorem

In the previous discussion we calculated the probability that a person with a positive ELISA had HIV antibodies, given known data about the prevalence of antibodies and the characteristics of the test. However, we had to take a roundabout route by calculating a new contingency table (Table 4-10) and then working out the appropriate values. There is an algebraic shortcut, called **Bayes's theorem**, that permits this calculation directly. To do the calculation, we will also introduce the following new symbols that frequently appear in the epidemiologic literature:

$$P(D) = \text{Probability of disease before the test}$$
$$= \text{Prevalence} = 0.2 \text{ percent}$$
$$P(T^+ \mid D) = \text{Probability of positive test given the disease}$$
$$= \text{Sensitivity} = 98.0 \text{ percent}$$
$$P(T^+ \mid \bar{D}) = \text{Probability of positive test given no disease}$$
$$= (1 - \text{Sensitivity}) = 0.8 \text{ percent}$$
$$P(T^- \mid D) = \text{Probability of negative test given the disease}$$
$$= (1 - \text{Sensitivity}) = 2.0 \text{ percent}$$
$$P(T^- \mid \bar{D}) = \text{Probability of negative test given no disease}$$
$$= \text{Sensitivity} = 99.2 \text{ percent}$$

According to Bayes' theorem, the probability of disease given a positive test, P(D I T+) (i.e., the positive predictive value), is as follows:

$$P(D \mid T^+) = \frac{P(D) \times P(T^+ \mid D)}{P(D) \times P(T^+ \mid D) + [1.0 - P(D)] \times P(T^+ \mid \bar{D})}$$
$$= \frac{0.2 \times 98}{(0.2 \times 98) + (0.8 \times 99.8)} = \frac{19.6}{99.4} = 19.7 \text{ percent}$$

A similar calculation could be done to get the negative predictive value.

Bayes's theorem can also be used in an iterative fashion. If we had a situation involving a series of laboratory tests, we could now calculate the posttest probability for the second, third, and subsequent tests. In each case, we would use the calculated posttest probability from the previous test as the pretest probability for the calculation of the next test.

Receiver Operating Characteristic Curves

One measure that is frequently used for evaluating the effectiveness of diagnostic systems is the **receiver operating characteristic (ROC)** curve. Particularly popular in radiology, it has roots in electrical engineering and psychophysics.

Imagine a laboratory test that has continuous values, such as cardiac enzymes, and consider the problem of attempting to find an appropriate cut-point where any value above the point is considered a positive (i.e., indicative of myocardial infarction) and any point below is considered negative or normal. If we set the point too high, we will miss a number of mild myocardial infarctions but will avoid false positives. Conversely, a point set too low will catch all the myocardial infarctions at the cost of filling cardiac care unit beds with normal (nonmyocardial infarction) patients. This situation is illustrated in Figure 4-1.

As we move the cut-point from right to left, we will initially pick up true positives and few false positives. However, as we pass the center of the myocardial infarction distribution, the rate of pickup of the false positives will increase and the true positives will decrease to the point that nearly all the increase is false positives. Plotting the true positive rate on the Y-axis and the false positive rate on the X-axis, we generate the ROC curve, as in Figure 4-2.

The ROC curve has some interesting features. First, we note that a perfect test would pick up only true positives at first, then after the true positive rate is 100%, only false positives; this describes a curve going vertically along the Y-axis and then horizontally along the top. Conversely, a useless test picks up both true and false positives at the same rate and traces out a line at 45°. The extent to which the ROC curve "crowds the corner" is a measure of the value of the test. This is measured by the area between the curve and the 45° line. Second, the best cutoff to minimize overall error rates occurs at the point nearest the upper left-hand corner, obtained by drawing a 45° tangent just touching the curve. A little geometry (measuring down and

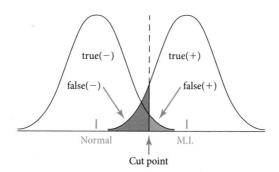

Figure 4-1. Determining the cut-point of a test for myocardial infarction (MI).

Figure 4-2. Receiver operating characteristic (ROC) curve.

across from the top left corner) shows that this is the point where the false positive and false negative rates are equal. In Figure 4-2, this corresponds to the point labeled 7/8, meaning that scores of 1 through 7 are considered to be normal, and 8 and above are abnormal. Displaying the data this way therefore permits a rational selection of the cutoff. Later we'll discuss situations where we may want to use some other cut-point. The advantage of the ROC approach is that it permits a clear separation between the intrinsic value of the test, as captured in the area under the curve, and the errors associated with an inappropriate choice of cutoff.

Moving the Cut-Point

As we've said, we minimize the rate of false positives and false negative when we use the cut-point that's closest to the upper left corner. But, that doesn't mean that we always want to use that cutoff. There are some situations where we can tolerate a high false positive rate, but false negatives can result in a significant problems. For example, we don't want to miss any units of donated blood that may have hepatitis-C or HIV floating around, so we would lower the cut-point to detect these. In other situations, it would be costly to have false positives. Professional and graduate schools, for example, have far more applicants than openings, and admitting people who will ultimately fail "wastes" slots that could have been used for people who would have passed, so the cut-point is raised to minimize this possibility.

Needless to say, these moves have costs associated with them. Those for screening blood are relatively low, as it would involve only unnecessarily throwing away some blood. Other times, the costs are much higher. Telling a person he or she may have hepatitis-C or HIV would be devastating news and could result in psychological sequelae from the labeling itself. In situations such as this, it would be best to follow up the first test with another one that has very high specificity in order to weed out the false positives before informing the person.

Accuracy

As yet we have not considered any measure of the overall accuracy of the test. One approach that is straightforward is to simply sum up the numbers on the diagonal of the table, cells A and D, and place them over the total of all cells. Let's use the data from our two AIDS examples (Tables 4-9 and 4-10).

The overall accuracy of the test, based on data from Table 4-9, is (498 + 488)/1000 = 98.6%. For the lower prevalence situation in Table 4-10, the accuracy is (1960 + 990,016)/1,000,000 = 99.198%. Even though the test is much less useful in the low prevalence case, the accuracy has improved because the huge numbers of true negatives have predominated in the calculation of accuracy. Because of the possibility of misleading results from this approach, most assessments of accuracy are performed by correcting for chance agreement using a statistic called Cohen's Kappa.

Chance Correction Using Cohen's Kappa

As we have just seen, the likelihood of agreement between a test result and a "gold standard" is affected by the prevalence of disease. In the extreme case we could consider the application of a clinical sign, right-handedness, to a classical "disease" of Victorian times—self-pollution, or masturbation. Right-handed people are in the majority with approximately 90% of the population. If we are in a population where everyone does "it," the test will be right 90% of the time without conveying any information whatsoever.

To avoid this trap, it is desirable to correct for chance agreement. Taking a little less extreme example, consider the data in Table 4-11, which predict depression as diagnosed by expert interview using Diagnostic and

Table 4-11
Prediction of Depression from Test Results

Test Results	Depression Present	Depression Absent	
Positive	18 (A)	7 (B)	25
Negative	12 (C)	63 (D)	75
	30	70	100

Statistical Manual of Mental Disorders-IV (DSM-IV) criteria from a self-completed questionnaire.

The accuracy, as determined before, is $(A + D)/N = (18 + 63)/100 = 81\%$. What agreement would we expect by chance? Chance means that there is, in fact, no association between the two variables. Consider first the A cell. We know that on the average, 30% of all people in the sample have depression, or 30 people. If there is no association between the two variables, we would expect that the same proportion of people with and without depression would have a positive test, simply equal to the overall proportion of positive tests, or 25%. So by chance, 25% of the 30 depressed people, or 7.5 people, would be in cell A. Similarly, there should be 75% of the nondepressed people, or 52.5 people, in cell D. The agreement expected by chance is $(7.5 + 52.5)/100 = 60\%$. We actually observed 81%. It's not necessary to figure out the numbers in cells B and C because we don't use them in the calculation. The chance corrected agreement, called **Kappa**, is defined as follows:

$$\text{Kappa} = \frac{\text{Observed agreement} - \text{Agreement by chance}}{1.0 - \text{Agreement by chance}} = \frac{0.81 - 0.60}{1.0 - 0.60}$$
$$= 0.21 / 0.40 = 0.525$$

As a result, the agreement corrected for chance has been reduced from 81% to 53%.

Now that we've developed a new diagnostic test, determined its properties (sensitivity, specificity, positive and negative predictive values), and have chosen the best cut-point using ROC analysis, why not put it to use, by giving it to everyone who's alive; in other words, shouldn't we use it to screen the population? After all, people are now getting gift certificates to have full-body CAT or MRI scans done for their birthdays. As we'll see, it may be better to give them another plaid tie or a bottle of perfume.

The rationale behind screening and early detection is shown in Figure 4-3. It's assumed that without it, people won't know that they have anything wrong with them until clinical signs appear, by which time it may be harder to treat the problem, or too late to do anything about it. Screening, though, would detect the problem earlier, while it is still in its pre-clinical stage, allowing for an earlier intervention that returns to the person to health and happiness. In oncology, where abnormal tissues are assigned to various stages, this is called a **stage shift**; that is, picking up a problem at an earlier stage of its development. However, screening is based on two assumptions: (1) that the natural history of whatever is detected is that it will progress to become a major problem; and (2) that a treatment exists that is effective.

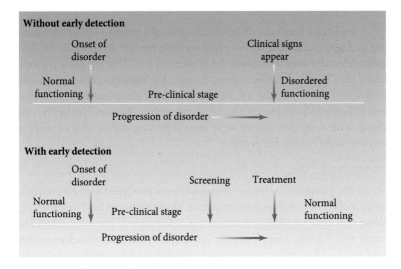

Figure 4-3. Supposed history of a disorder without (top) and with (bottom) screening.

Length Bias

One of the (many) problems associated with screening for prostate cancer is that a large number of "abnormalities" that are detected are very slow-growing and would not lead to any problems if left to their own devices. That is, the men in whom these lesions are seen will have been dead for many years from other causes before these growths would have done anything nasty to them. This is called the **length bias**—the detection of less-aggressive "diseases" that won't actually harm you. In fact, in one study involving 71,000 men, the mortality rate was the same in the screened and unscreened groups. Length bias is a particular problem under two conditions: when the disorder is a heterogeneous one, with some forms progressing quickly and aggressively, and other forms just quietly sitting there minding their own business; and when many people have detectable but undiagnosed problems for a long time. The one advantage of early screening in this situation is that it makes survival statistics look better—we've increased the number of people known to have the disease who don't die from it. Isn't medicine marvelous? Not really; we haven't touched the number of people who get better, just the number of people who are labeled.

The same thing happens when diagnostic tests become more sensitive and better able to pick up smaller lesions. The introduction of ultrasound and fine-needle aspiration led to a 2.4-fold increase in the incidence of thyroid cancer between 1973 and 2002. However, the mortality rate from this "disease" remained unchanged over the same interval.

Lead-Time Bias

A **lead-time bias** exists when we do pick up a potentially life-threatening problem earlier, but there's precious little we can do about it. All that early detection does is increase the amount of time that the poor patients know they have a disorder. Again, though, the statistics look better—the proportion of people who are alive 5 years after diagnosis has increased, and it looks like people are living longer with it. Not really; they're still dying at the same age, and all we've done is prolong the number of years of anxiety about having the problem.

Compliance Bias

In the previous chapter, we discussed biases that affect who enters trials, and the effect of compliance on outcomes. The same things exist in screening: those who agree to undergo it are compliant volunteers. They are healthier to begin with than the general population, and their inclusion makes screening look good—people who are screened live longer, but it has nothing to do with the screening, and everything to do with who they are.

Other Problems with Screening

Screening, especially for low-prevalence conditions, can lead to other problems. One immutable law of nature is that when the prevalence of a disorder is low, the false positive rate is high. For example, one study that used fetal monitoring to detect cerebral palsy had a false positive rate of 99.8%. This results in a number of adverse consequences. First, there's the effect of labeling itself. Once they were told they had hypertension, men's absenteeism increased, even though their physical state hadn't changed; and healthy children who were wrongly told they had heart murmurs had more "illness behavior" than children who were unaware that they actually did have a murmur. Second, the health care system has trouble enough managing the people who actually are ill. Imagine the chaos when it becomes flooded with newly detected "cases," many of whom either don't have the disorder, or can't be effectively treated. Finally, there are the dangers of the diagnostic test itself (e.g., X-ray mammography) or the biopsies used to rule out the disorder.

When to Screen

Let's put all of these advantages and caveats together to determine when it does and doesn't make sense to screen. One set of criteria, proposed by Cuckle and Ward, looks at the disease, the test, and the policy. The disease should be medically important and be clearly defined; and it should have a known prognosis, prevalence, and treatment. The test should be safe, reliable, and valid. Finally, with regard to policy, the screening program must be cost-effective; there must be existing facilities to diagnose and treat the disorder; and what to do after a positive test result must be agreed up and acceptable. Well, there go most screening programs.

MEASUREMENT WITH CONTINUOUS VARIABLES

Historically, epidemiology was concerned with the distribution in time and place of disease epidemics; in more recent times, clinical epidemiology has focused on the testing of therapies directed to prolonging life by reducing the incidence of such catastrophic events as heart attacks and strokes. In these situations, the unit of analysis is the case of disease or death, and measurement issues focus on the verification of presence or absence of disease.

However, physicians and epidemiologists are increasingly coming to recognize that for many diseases, there is little to be gained in *quantity* of life from foreseeable advances in biomedicine, and there is much more potential for gain in *quality* of life. Innovations such as palliative care and geriatric medicine are explicitly not directed to the cure of disease or extension of life; rather, they are an attempt to improve the quality of life.

From the perspective of epidemiology, research in this area presents new measurement challenges. The measurement of quality of life is a new science; different methods proliferate and seldom yield the same results. There is possibly more error of measurement than might be expected in categorical measures like diagnosis. Conventional approaches to evaluation of measures, such as comparison with a "gold standard," are inapplicable because no such criterion currently exists and no clinical equivalent of the autopsy or biopsy will ever be available. Epidemiologists must acquire new skills, borrowed from such disciplines as psychology, education, and economics, to understand and contribute to the development of these measures.

With rare exceptions, these outcomes are based on continuous measurement, originating in rating scales or checklists completed by observers or patients. Approaches to the measurement of association with these measures involve unfamiliar concepts like reliability and construct validity. Usually analysis is conducted using parametric statistics, which assume an interval level of measurement and normal (bell-shaped) distributions. This section briefly reviews some of these concepts. We are not trying to be comprehensive; instead, we will recommend additional readings for readers who wish to venture further.

Measures of Association

To examine the issues of measurement with continuous variables, we will use an example from rheumatology. The issues here are prototypical of the issues we raised in the beginning of this discussion. The diseases of rheumatology—rheumatoid arthritis, osteoarthritis, ankylosing spondylitis, and lupus—are rarely fatal but often are severely incapacitating because they inflict pain, deformity, and dysfunction on their victims. To examine the efficacy of their therapies, rheumatologists have developed a large number of measures of disease severity. Some emerge from the laboratory, such as erythrocyte sedimentation rate and rheumatoid factor, but appear to have little relationship with clinical measures of function. Some appear to be "objective" clinical descriptions of disease process, such as counts of involved joints or erosion counts (from observations of bone erosions on hand radiographs) and walk times. On closer scrutiny, however, these objective descriptions appear to have a great deal of variation among observers and relatively little relationship with measures of the patient's function. Finally, some measures are based on the patients' own assessment of their function and health and run the gamut from a simple 10-cm line (called a visual analog scale, presumably to obscure its simplicity) on which the patient puts a mark to indicate the perceived health, to indices of function containing tens or hundreds of questions.

To make sense of this potpourri, it is essential to review empirical evidence that the measures are doing what was intended by their makers. When these questions are examined, the evidence falls into two broad classes. The researcher assessing **reliability** asks whether the measures are giving the same answer over different situations (e.g., different observers or the same observer on two occasions separated by a short time interval). When we study **validity**, we are asking what conclusions we can correctly draw about the person based on his or her score on the scale. Can we truly say that a person who scores higher on a quality of life index has a better quality than someone who scores lower?

Because the measures are continuous, we cannot simply place the data into a 2 × 2 table as we used before. (We could do this, but the shoehorn act comes at an awful cost of loss of information; for example, any height greater than 5'6" [168 cm] is classified as tall.) Instead we must measure the degree to which an individual who is high on one measure or occasion is high on a second measure or occasion and the converse. The methods to develop these measures are explored further in the next discussions.

Pearson Correlation

By far the most common measure of association for continuous variables is the **Pearson product-moment correlation**. It was invented in the early 1900s by one of the founders of modern statistics. The correlation is based on the idea of fitting the data by a straight line, as illustrated in Figure 4-4.

The Pearson correlation is a number between −1 and + 1. It equals 0 if there is no relationship and 1 if there is a perfect linear (straight line) relationship. There is one minor addition: if the slope is negative, that is, if the joint count decreases with increasing sedimentation rate, the correlation is preceded by a minus sign. Therefore a perfect negative relationship has a correlation of −1. Pearson correlations of various sizes are pictured in Figure 4-5.

As you can see, the more the individual points deviate from the straight line, the lower the correlation. With a perfect correlation (+1 or −1), all the points fall on the line. It should be evident from Figure 4-5 that a correlation

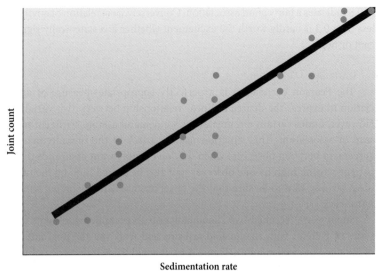

Figure 4-4. Association between erythrocyte sedimentation rate and a measure of active joints in patients with rheumatoid arthritis.

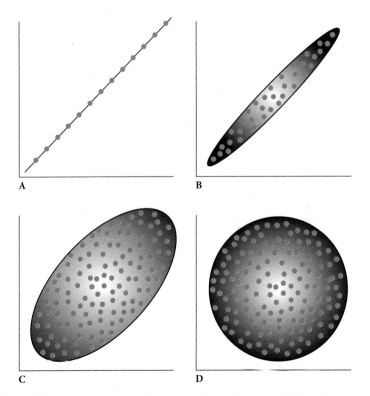

Figure 4-5. Correlations of various sizes. **A**, r = 1; **B**, r = 0.9; 9, **C**, r = 0.5; **D**, r = 0.

of 0.8 indicates a fairly good association. Conversely, a correlation of anything less than 0.3 is hardly worth the excitement whether it is statistically significant or not.

Intraclass Correlation

The Pearson correlation is a perfectly appropriate measure of association to express the degree of linear relationship between two variables. However, under certain circumstances we demand a more stringent measure of association. This situation usually arises in the measurement of agreement between observers when we don't simply want assurance that a patient scoring high by one observer will also be scored high by the other observer; we want to be sure that the observers are actually giving similar numbers.

Suppose we recruited two rheumatologists to examine hand joints on a series of patients with rheumatoid arthritis and work out the total number of inflamed or swollen joints (Figure 4-6). It could happen that one observer set much lower thresholds for what he or she chose to call "inflamed" than the other, so that for every patient the total was exactly two more (i.e., if one observer said 12 joints, the second said 10, and if one said 4, the other said 2).

The Pearson correlation simply demands that there is a strong association between the raters—the highest scoring patients for Observer 1 are also the highest for Observer 2, and the lowest for Observer 1 are the lowest for Observer 2. Because this is the case and the points all lie exactly on a straight line, we would get a Pearson correlation of +1. However, by most standards the agreement is not great because the observers never give the patient the same count.

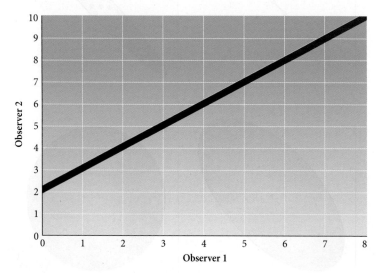

Figure 4-6. The number of hand joints judged as inflamed by two rheumatologists for various patients.

To get around this problem, the Pearson correlation has been replaced in most circles by the **intraclass correlation** (**ICC**). The ICC is still expressed as a number between 0 and 1; however, the ICC measures not only the *association* between the raters but also the *agreement*.

Although much is made of the differences between association and agreement and the relative advantages of the ICC over the Pearson correlation, in most real-world situations the major variability in the data is from apparently random error. Under these circumstances the two measures give identical results. Furthermore, if we treat a 2 × 2 table as a series of points having values of (1,1), (0,0), (1,0), or (0,1), the ICC and Kappa yield identical results. For once, we can get convergence among differing approaches.

Reliability

Reliability is, as we indicated, a measure of the extent to which a measure is reproducible, or gives the same results, over different situations (e.g., different observers or different days). However, this reproducibility is defined in a special way by comparing the variability across situations (error variance) with the true variability among patients (patient variance). The reliability coefficient is defined as follows:

$$\text{Reliability} = \frac{\text{Variance caused by patients}}{\text{Variance caused by patients} + \text{Error variance}}$$

In other words, the reliability expresses the proportion of the variability in the measures that is caused by true variability among patients. The implication of this definition is that if the patients we are studying are truly homogeneous with respect to the attribute of interest, the reliability of the measure will be near 0; conversely, if there is great variability among patients, there will likely be higher reliability. The reliability is a measure of the extent to which we can *differentiate* among patients on a particular attribute.

Although this definition is a bit hard for egalitarian folks to accept, it rests on the simple premise that the goal of measurement is to distinguish among people on a particular attribute. If all the people in the population have the same value of a particular quantity, why bother to measure it? Simply assume that the next person will have that value too.

It is not too difficult to demonstrate that the phenomenon is completely analogous to the discussion about the effect of prevalence on the performance of a diagnostic test. Reliability is like the chance corrected accuracy of a test. If the prevalence of disease drops, this is analogous to the patient population becoming more similar, and the reliability of the continuous measure and the accuracy of the test both fall.

There are some other terms usually associated with reliability, most of which are self-explanatory. **Interobserver** reliability examines the degree of agreement among different observers. **Test-retest** reliability involves administering a test or measure to a group of patients on two different occasions and examining the correlation. **Split-halves** reliability is used in longer tests and involves splitting the test items into two halves at random and examining the correlations between subscores from the two halves of the test.

There are a number of other specific forms of reliability, but this should give you the idea.

Validity

Having shown that a measure is reliable, it remains to be shown what the scores actually mean. Sometimes this is straightforward and uncontroversial; for example, to show that a mercury manometer is measuring blood pressure validly, we can simply compare blood pressure values obtained in this way with direct measures of arterial blood pressure.

More often, though, the situation is not so obvious. How do you know that your new measure is really assessing quality of life, anxiety, locus of control, or whatever? Even more critically, what does a score of X on a certain measure tell us about the person? Is a score of Y on a depression inventory well within the normal range, or something that we should be worried about? We have now entered the world of validity. Validity used to be defined as demonstrating that the scale is measuring what we think it measures. More recently, though, it has been redefined as telling us what conclusions we can safely draw about a person knowing his or her test score. Like reliability, validity is not an intrinsic property of the scale, but is rather an interaction of the test, the person taking it, and the circumstances. Tests that are valid for one group of people under some circumstances (e.g., middle-class males applying for a job) may not be valid for other people in different situations (lower-SES people being assessed for the courts).

Also in light of recent thinking, we will not talk of different "types" of validity. All of validity testing is now seen as part of **construct validity** (which we'll define in a bit). Rather, there are different *ways* of assessing construct validity. Thus, we will talk about *content validation* (i.e., a process) instead of *content validity* (that is, a type of validity).

Face and Content Validation

Face validation asks whether the scale looks, "on the face of it," to measure the construct we're interested in. It's usually done by asking a group of experts and patients if the scale as a whole appear to be relevant. Face validation doesn't make the scale better, just more acceptable to users. **Content validation** tries to ensure that (a) all aspects of the construct have been tapped, and (b) the scale doesn't measure irrelevant things. This is done a number of ways, starting with a thorough review of the literature and other scales. We can also ask patients and experts in the field what they think would be relevant questions to ask. Once a preliminary draft of a questionnaire is developed, it's sent to 5 to 10 experts who are asked to rate each item on its relevance to the construct, and to indicate whether any part of the construct has been short-changed.

Although these steps are fairly time consuming, they are relatively weak tests of validity, because they rely solely on people's judgment. Also, the experts whom we ask to evaluate the scales are usually our colleagues, who often share the same understanding of the construct as we do. (Only small-minded people would say they have the same biases.)

Criterion Validation

As we indicated, measures of validity based on expert judgments are regarded in general as weak tests of validity. Perhaps the strongest approach to validity is the assessment of **criterion validation**, which involves comparison with a "gold standard." In turn, this is divided into two forms that differ only in time. If the comparison is made at the same time (i.e., both measures are administered together), the approach is called **concurrent validation**. If the measure is used to predict future status, such as confirmation of a disease at autopsy or admission to hospital, it is call **predictive validation**. The index of criterion validation is most often a correlation coefficent between the scores on the new test and on the old (or predicted) one.

The comparison of blood pressure reading with a mercury sphygmomanometer with arterial blood pressures is an example that highlights both the use of a "gold standard" and the reason for developing a new measure, namely, reduced cost or risk. However, such true "gold standards" are difficult to come by, and one is frequently left in the situation of comparing the new measure with another better accepted but arguably inferior measure of the same attribute. One example of this is the measurement of depression. Although new measures proliferate, nearly all are compared with one of two scales—the Beck Depression Inventory or the Center for Epidemiological Studies-Depression (CES-D) scale. Because both standards are short and cheap, the only reason to develop a new measure is to make it better; however, this is difficult to prove by simply comparing with existing measures. Under these circumstances the expected correlation of two measures should be high, but one would not anticipate correlations too close to unity; if it were nearly 1.0, the two tests are measuring almost exactly the same thing and there is little reason to develop the new one.

Construct Validation

For historical reasons, the term **construct validation** has two overlapping meanings. First, as we said earlier, all research that tries to determine the meaning of the scale and the interpretation of its scores can be thought of as construct validational studies. But, the older use of the term refers to types of studies not subsumed under face, content, or criterion validation (confusing, right?). Used in this latter sense, construct validation is done when there is no gold standard, so we can't rely on criterion validation. Instead of testing the relationship between measures, we fall back on our understanding of the construct and make predictions about how the scale should perform under different circumstances.

For example, if we were developing a measure of quality of life for patients with rheumatoid arthritis, we could hypothesize a number of findings. One would be that the scale is strongly related to measures of functioning, such as morning stiffness or walking time, but that it is not related to measures of disease process like joint count or sedimentation rate. Another hypothesis is that scores should improve after the patients begins treatment; or that patients who are in hospital because of their arthritis should have lower scores than out-patients. Every study that supports a hypothesis strengthens the validation of the scale.

It is evident that in the construct validity game there is no single study or hypothesis that clinches the case. Some hypotheses will be right and some will be wrong. Rather, the judgment of validity depends on the *weight* of the evidence being in the expected direction.

Measurement Bias

In the previous section on research methodology (see Chapter 3) we described how incorrect conclusions may result from design flaws. Biases such as the Berkson's bias and Neyman bias can yield estimates that are systematically higher or lower than the true value.

Unfortunately, research design errors are not the only source of bias. Large distortions can result from bias in measurement. There are innumerable sources of measurement bias; many psychologists have made careers out of cataloging how people can be induced to distort their estimates one way or another. One of the most disturbing examples derives from choices resembling the following: "You are responsible for the care of 100 patients who have a fatal disease. You are given a choice between two drugs: Drug A has a 60% chance of saving everyone; Drug B will save 60 of the 100 patients. Which will you choose?"

Under these circumstances, most subjects choose Drug B. However, the question can be framed in the logically equivalent way: "You are responsible for the care of 100 patients with a fatal disease. You are given a choice between two drugs. Drug A has 40% chance of killing all the patients. Drug B will result in the death of 40 of the 100 patients. Which will you choose?"

When the question is framed in this way, most respondents choose Drug A. Obviously, the way in which a question is asked can lead to radically different responses. There are many other ways that data can be willingly or unwillingly distorted by unsuspecting investigators. Our purpose will be served by illustrating a few.

However, before we illustrate a few different kinds of bias, let's distinguish between two concepts—bias and random error. **Bias** is a *systematic* deviation from the correct value of a particular variable. The effect of bias is to distort the estimate of the variable, for example, to increase the sample mean or decrease the prevalence of some trait. In **random error**, on the other hand, there is also a deviation from the true value, but because it is random the deviation sometimes adds to the estimate and sometimes takes from it. In the long run (i.e., with a lot of subjects) these deviations cancel out each other. The effect is to increase the variability of the scores, but random error does not affect the estimate of the variable. For this reason, random error can be dealt with by statistics. Because bias is a *consistent* distortion from the true value, it cannot be corrected by any statistical manipulation and thus is more insidious.

Social Desirability Bias

Personality psychologists now routinely include a **social desirability** scale in many of their measures. The notion is that people, when asked sensitive questions about, for example, alcohol consumption or sexual practices, will consciously or unconsciously bias their responses toward the socially acceptable answer. If the bias is deliberate and conscious, it is called "faking good," and if unconscious, "social desirability." In either case, the results are the same—an underestimate of the true prevalence of undersirable behaviors.

Several techniques have been developed to detect the presence of social desirability and to fix it if present. Many psychological scales contain imbedded social desirability scales; for example, only saints can truthfully answer "true" to the statement "I have never stolen anything." Alternatively, methods such as the random response technique are designed to elicit better measures of the prevalance of unacceptable behaviors.

C.R.A.P. DETECTORS
C.R.A.P. Detector IV-1

Question. An investigation of the usefulness of exercise electrocardiograms (ECG) was conducted using patients who had been admitted to a coronary care unit. The ECG was compared with findings from coronary angiography—an expensive and risky procedure. For obvious reasons the researchers had difficulty recruiting a large number of "normal" subjects to undergo angiography. So they took 80 men off the street, performed ECGs on them (which were normal of course), assumed that they would have normal angiograms, and added them to the negative ECG-negative angiogram category. The results looked good indeed: sensitivity was 64% and specificity was 93%. Subsequent applications of exercise ECGs in ambulatory settings have shown that it is not what it was cracked up to be and shows a sensitivity of only 33%. Why does the discrepancy exist?

Answer. The authors did two things to ensure that the results would look favorable. First, the positive cases were chosen from a highly select group of men in coronary care units with confirmed cardiac disease, so they were more extreme than the usual suspected arteriosclerotics. Second, the initial study had too high a prevalence of disease. By including the "normal" volunteers and, better still, assuming that they had normal angiograms, they succeeded in messing the base rates in their favor.

Beware the "sample samba." By dancing around with prevalence or by selecting extreme groups (e.g., physical education students and 70-year-olds on their third myocardial infarction), anyone can make any test in the world look good.

C.R.A.P. Detector IV-2

Question. A recent reanalysis was conducted of the Blair et al. National Cancer Institute study of the occupational effects of formaldehyde on cancer. They were unable to show any significant relationship between formaldehyde level and lung cancer but did demonstrate a relationship between job class and cancer. They concluded that the retrospective measurement of formaldehyde was too crude and that blue-collar workers suffered more lung cancer as a result of occupational exposure to formaldehyde. The study was not published (thank goodness!). Why?

Answer. The measurement of formaldehyde level may have been crude, but the use of job class as a surrogate for exposure ignores the many other variables that go along with job class. First, blue-collar workers smoke more, and smoking causes lung cancer. Second, folks of a "lower" social class suffer more disease of all types and live shorter lives than "upper"- class folks.

Correlation is not equal to causation. (See Chapter 5.)

C.R.A.P. Detector IV-3

Question. In a study of the causes of cervical cancer one potential cause under investigation was whether the man was circumcised. The researchers approached 166 men and asked whether they were circumcised. This was then confirmed by a physical examination. Of the 44 men who said they were, 21 (48%) were not, and of the 122 men who said they were not circumcised, 50 (40%) were! Don't men know whether they are circumcised?

Answer. Self-report may be a lousy lab test. If an investigator is using self-report data, there should be some assurance (other than faith!) that the data are valid.

C.R.A.P. Detector IV-4

Question. For approximately 2 decades, patient management problems (PMPs) have been used as a component in the licensure examination used to license physicians in Canada and the United States. These are written simulations of a patient on which the candidate selects options on history, physical, laboratory, and management and is rewarded (or punished) on the basis of the good options he or she selected and harmful options he or she avoided. Many studies demonstrated that candidates believed the method to be lifelike (face validation), and care was taken to ensure that they were medically accurate (content validation). They have also been used as a measure of problem-solving skills. This was confirmed by a low correlation of PMP results with tests of knowledge, which suggested that they were measuring "something else" (construct validation). Can PMPs be considered to be good predictors of physician performance?

Answer. Recent studies showed a low reliability of the scores, which suggests that the "something else" they were measuring was simply noise. Other studies showed that candidates do approximately twice as much of everything (such as ordering lab tests) on the written problem as they do in real life. Both licensing bodies have subsequently dropped the requirement for performance on PMPs.

Face and content validation are poor substitutes for empirical forms of validity. Anyone can recruit some friends who will like his or her measure. The best test of validity is criterion-related validity. All others are relatively weak approximations.

REFERENCES

Issues in Choosing a Measure

Sears FW, Zemansky MW: *College physics: mechanics, heat and sound*, Reading, MA, 1952, Addison-Wesley.

Measurement with Categorical Variables

Doll R, Peto R: *The causes of cancer*, Oxford, 1981, Oxford University Press.
Laupacis A, Sackett DL, Roberts, RS: An assessment of clinically useful measures of the consequences of treatment, *N Engl J Med* 318:1728–1733, 1988.
Lipid Research Clinics Program: The Lipid Research Clinics coronary prevention trials results, *JAMA* 251:351–374, 1984.

Muntoni S: Cholesterol-lowering drugs for primary prevention: the WOSCOP Study. *Pharmacol Res* 35:169–170, 1997.

Walter SD: Choice of effect measure for epidemiological data, *J Clin Epidemiol* 53:931–939, 2000.

Wynder EL, Graham EA: Tobacco smoking as a possible etiologic factor in broncho-genic carcinoma: a study of 684 proved cases, *JAMA* 143:329–336, 1950.

Diagnostic Tests

Cohen J: Weighted kappa: nominal scale agreement with provision for scaled dis-agreement or partial credit, *Psychol Bull* 70:213–222, 1968.

Gibertini M, Brandenburg N, Retzlaff P: The operating characteristics of the Millon Clinical Multiaxial Inventory, *J Pers Assess* 50:554–567, 1986.

Kraemer HC: *Evaluating medical tests: objective and quantitative guidelines*, Newbury Park, Calif., 1992, Sage.

Lusted L: *Medical decision making*, Springfield, 1968, CC Thomas.

Meehl PE, Rosen A: Antecedent probability and the efficiency of psychometric signs, patterns, or cutting scores, *Psychol Bull* 52:194–216, 1955.

National Cancer Institute of Canada: *Canadian cancer statistics*, Toronto, 1995, NCIC.

Petricoin EF, Ardekani AM, Hitt BA, et al.: Use of proteomic patterns in serum to identify ovarian cancer. *Lancet* 359:572–577, 2002.

Polesky HF: Serologic testing to human immunodeficiency virus, *Morb Mortal Wkly Rep* 36:833, 1986.

Screening

Alderman MH, Charlson ME, Melcher LA: Labelling and absenteeism: the Massachusetts Mutual experience, *Clin Invest Med* 4:165–171, 1981.

Bergman AB, Stamm SJ: The morbidity of cardiac nondisease in schoolchildren, *N Engl J Med* 276:1008–1013, 1967.

Coley CM, Barry MJ, Fleming C, Mulley AG: Clinical guideline: part 1: early detec-tion of prostate cancer: Part I. prior probability and effectiveness of tests, *Ann Int Med* 126:394-406, 1997.

Concato J,.Wells CK, Horwitz RI, et al.: The effectiveness of screening for prostate cancer: a nested case-control study, *Arch Int Med* 166:38–43, 2006.

Cuckle HS, Ward NJ: Principles of screening. In Wald NJ, Leck I, editors: *Antenatal and prenatal screening*, Oxford, 1984, Oxford University Press.

Davies L, Welch HG: Increasing incidence of thyroid cancer in the United States, 1973–2002, *JAMA* 295:2164–2167, 2006.

Gann PH, Hennekens CH, Stampfer MJ: A prospective evaluation of plasma pros-tate-specific antigen for detection of prostatic cancer, *JAMA*. 273:289–294, 1995.

Gerber GS, Thompson IM, Thisted R, Chodak GW: Disease-specific survival following routine prostate cancer screening by digital rectal examination. *JAMA*.269:61–64, 1993.

Nelson KB, Dambrosia JM, Ting TY, Grether JK: Uncertain value of electronic fetal monitoring in predicting cerebral palsy, *New Engl J Med* 334:613–618, 1996.

Streiner DL: Diagnosing tests: using and misusing diagnostic and screening tests, *J Pers Assess* 81:209–219, 2003.

Measurement with Continuous Variables

American Psychological Association: *Standards for educational and psychological testing*, ed 3, Washington, DC, 1985, APA.

Crowne DP, Marlowe D: A new scale of social desirability independent of psychopathology, *J Consult Psychol* 24:349–354, 1960.

Eraker SA, Sox HC: Assessment of patients' preferences for therapeutic outcomes, *Med Decis Making* 1:29–39, 1981.

Warner SL: Randomized response: a survey technique for eliminating evasive answer bias, *J Am Stat Assoc* 60:63–69, 1965.

C.R.A.P. Detectors

Blair A: Mortality among workers exposed to formaldehyde, *J Natl Cancer Inst* 75:1039–1047, 1985.

Dunn JE, Buell P: Association of cervical cancer with circumcision of sexual partner, *J Natl Cancer Inst* 22:749–764, 1959.

Goldschlager N, Selzer A, Cohn K: Treadmill stress tests as indicators of presence and severity of coronary artery disease, *Ann Intern Med* 85:277–286, 1976.

McGuire CH, Babbott D: Simulation technique in the measurement of problem-solving skills, *J Educ Meas* 4:1–10, 1967.

TO READ FURTHER

Measurement with Categoric Variables

McMahon B, Pugh TF: *Epidemiology: principles and methods*, Boston, 1970, Little, Brown.

Diagnostic Tests

McNeil BJ, Hanley JA: Statistical approaches to the analysis of receiver operating characteristic (ROC) curves, *Med Decis Making* 4:137–150, 1984.

Sackett DL, Haynes RB, Tugwell P: *Clinical epidemiology: a basic science for clinical medicine*, Boston, 1985, Little, Brown.

Measurement with Continuous Variables

Anastasi A: *Psychological testing*, ed 5, New York, 1982, Macmillan.

Kahnemann D, Slovic P, Tversky A: *Judgment under uncertainty: heuristics and biases*, Cambridge, Cambridge University Press.

Norman GR, Streiner DL: *PDQ Statistics,* ed 3, Toronto, 2003, BC Decker.

Streiner DL, Norman, GR: *Health measurement scales: a practical guide to their development and use*, ed 4, Oxford, 2008, Oxford University Press.

5

Assessing Causation

In this chapter, we will look at how epidemiologists attempt to establish causation, that is, to decide whether factor A can possibly be the cause of disorder or state B. Perhaps the earliest rules for assessing causation were Koch's Postulates, which were set forth approximately a century ago for determining whether an infectious agent is the cause of a disease. These postulates assumed the following:

1. Every diseased person (or animal) must have the organism.
2. It must be possible to isolate the organism and grow it in a pure culture.
3. A susceptible host, when inoculated with the organism, must develop the disease.
4. The organism must be recoverable from the newly infected host.

Although these could easily be applied to acute infectious diseases, there are many situations in which the rules do not apply. Sir A. Bradford Hill proposed a variation of these criteria that covers a greater variety of situations, which has been used with little modification ever since. These nine criteria, listed in descending order of importance, are the following:

1. The **strength** of the association,
2. The **consistency** of the association,
3. Its **specificity**,
4. The **temporal** relationship,
5. The **biological** gradient,
6. Biological **plausibility**,
7. **Coherence**,
8. Evidence from **experimentation**, and
9. **Analogy**.

We will use these criteria to examine one theory of the etiology of multiple sclerosis (MS). In many ways, MS is an intriguing disease. One of the most puzzling aspects is its geographic distribution; the prevalence seems to be directly proportional to distance from the equator. The disorder is far more common in the northern parts of North America and the southern parts of Australia and New Zealand than it is in the tropics. However, just to make things a bit more interesting, MS is rare in Japan, a country at the same latitude as California.

A number of etiologic theories have been proposed that try to account for this distribution of MS. These have ranged from a genetic predisposition to the disorder, to dietary factors, to exposure, and to canine excrement. One group of theories holds that MS is caused by a viral agent, possibly even a slow virus (a class of viruses frequently invoked by researchers whenever the relationship between exposure and outcome is not readily apparent). In this chapter we will focus on one viral theory, exposure to the measles virus, to see whether it is a plausible explanation.

THE CRITERIA

Strength of Association

This criterion holds that the stronger the association between the supposed cause and the effect, the greater the chances are that a causal relationship exists. In this example, there should be a higher rate of multiple sclerosis among people who have been exposed to the measles virus than among those who have not been exposed. Conversely, measles antibody titers may be higher in MS patients than in people who do not have the disease.

The original data in this regard were tantalizing, but inconclusive (what is called the "So what else in new?" effect in epidemiology). Adams and Imagawa found that various measles antibody titers were higher in MS patients than in people without the disease. However, as can be seen in Table 5-1, the magnitude of the relationship wasn't too strong, although a trend is definitely present. But, people may have been looking in the wrong place. About 15 years later, Cook and his group used a fluorescent antibody method in the jejunal mucosa (that's the middle section of the small intestine) and found more conclusive evidence—antigens and complements were found in 18 of the 24 MS patients, but none of the controls. So, this argument was strengthened, but it led to other arguments—what was the virus doing in the gut?

Consistency of Association

The association between the suspected cause and the outcome should be seen across numerous studies, ideally by different research teams, in different settings, and under different circumstances. The larger the number of studies that demonstrate such a relationship, the stronger the evidence. There have

Table 5-1 Percentage of Subjects Greater Than/Less Than 32 on the Serum Dilution Test for Measles Virus

		MS Patients	Controls
Reciprocal of Serum Dilution	<32	64	86
	>32	36	14

From Adams JM, Imagawa D: Measles antibodies in multiple sclerosis, Proc Soc Exp Biol Med 111:562–566, 1962.

been approximately 35 such studies conducted since 1962, and higher titers of measles antibodies were found in MS patients in all but four of them. So this criterion would lend support to a causal hypothesis involving exposure to measles.

However, in and of itself, consistency does not *prove* association much less causation. (Indeed, none of the criteria proves causation; they can only be used either to strengthen or to weaken the case for it.) All of the studies can suffer from the same types of bias. For example, a number of studies showed that the use of conjugated estrogens was associated with a much higher risk of endometrial carcinoma. However, Horwitz and Feinstein pointed out that all of the studies suffered from the same type of sampling bias: women were identified on the basis of vaginal bleeding. Estrogens may cause bleeding, which leads to an intensive work-up during which the cancer is discovered. It is possible (indeed, they found it probable) that endometrial cancer is almost as prevalent in the general population, but women who did not take estrogens didn't have the symptom of vaginal bleeding, and so their cancer was not detected (see the discussion on subject selection biases in *Threats to Validity* in Chapter 3). When the bias was eliminated, the odds ratio dropped from 11.98 to 1.7, or in essence from a twelvefold risk of developing cancer for women who have used estrogens to less than a twofold risk.

Specificity of Association

Ideally, the cause should lead to only one outcome, and that outcome should result from that single cause (Figure 5-1). Unfortunately, life is rarely this simple. Obviously not everyone who gets measles later develops MS; measles can lead to a host of other adverse outcomes (including sterility), and it is possible that MS is multidetermined and has other causes (e.g., genetic predisposition, exposure to other viruses). In fact, Cook et al., who found

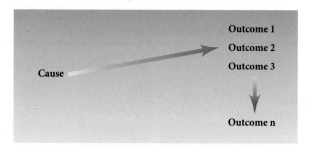

Figure 5-1. Ideal specificity of association.

measles viruses in the intestines of all MS patients they assessed, also found the parainfluenza virus and one associated with slow virus disease in animals. To use another example, obesity increases the risk not only for stroke but also for diabetes; however, both diabetes and stroke can arise from causes other than obesity.

When specificity does exist, it can be a powerful argument for causality. For example, the annual rate of malignant mesothelioma is extemely low, averaging fewer than 3 cases per million for men and approximately 1.4 cases per million for women. The incidence of mesothelioma among asbestos workers, however, is 100 to 200 times higher. It has also been estimated that there was exposure to asbestos in at least 85% percent of the mesothelioma cases; indeed, even this high figure may be an underestimate because families of asbestos workers are at risk through fibers brought home on clothing. It would seem from this evidence that there is a high degree of specificity because exposure to asbestos is found in nearly all cases of mesothelioma.

Thus if there is specificity of association, it strengthens the case for causality. However, a lack of specifity does not necessarily weaken the case.

Temporality of Association

For factor A to cause outcome B, A must precede B (Figure 5-2). That is, the person must have been exposed to the putative cause before the onset of the disorder. Although this criterion may appear so self-evident that it hardly bears mentioning, it is indeed difficult to establish in many cases, especially for chronic conditions with long latency periods. In the case of MS and measles it is obvious that the *clinical onset* of measles precedes that of MS; however, it would have to be shown that MS did not have a long, insidious onset that may have begun *before* the person contracted measles.

To use a different example, a number of studies demonstrated that a low serum cholesterol level was associated with a higher risk of cancer, which led some to postulate that a low cholesterol level somehow results in cancer. Recently, however, Dyer showed that the more likely explanation is that undetected cancer leads to a lowering of the cholesterol level. Thus the

Figure 5-2. Temporality of association.

purported "cause," cholesterol level, may actually occur *after* what was supposed to be the "effect," cancer.

One field particularly prone to problems in interpreting temporality is psychiatry, especially with respect to those studies that try to uncover family patterns that predispose people to major disorders. Because many problems manifest themselves only when the patient is in his or her 20s or 30s, the vast majority of studies use either retrospective case-series or case-control designs. The assumption made is that any family dynamics uncovered were present before the onset of the disorder. For example, the supposed etiology of early infantile autism was once thought to be the emotional coldness and withdrawal of the parents, especially of the mother. However, later studies indicated that these attributes were more likely the parents' reactions to an unresponsive infant, rather than the cause, thereby supporting what parents have long maintained: insanity is inherited—we get it from our children.

There is another point to keep in mind when thinking about time; there must be sufficient time for the exposure to have had an observable effect. If we're looking for a link between extremely low birth weight (< 1,000 grams) and cardiovascular disease (the "Barker Hypothesis"), for instance, it doesn't make sense to examine 2-month old neonates; the effects likely won't be noticeable until the kids are at least in their 20s.

One real example came from the UFFI (urea formaldehyde foam insulation) debacle of the 1980s. Concurrent with the perceived problems of UFFI, a study of rats showed that at high formaldehyde doses, they got nasal cancer. Regrettably, the television program, 20/20, smelling a scandal, found someone who had installed UFFI in his house a year or two earlier, and whose wife had subsequently died of nasal cancer. The grief-stricken widower openly expressed his sorrow that his decision to install UFFI killed his wife. Problem was that the time between installation and death was only a couple of years; not enough time for cancer to develop. But it had the desired effect anyway; a public outcry about yet another environmental "hazard." It also proves the dictum that the plural of "anecdote" is not "data."

Biological Gradient

The biological gradient, or dose-response relationship, states that if more exposure leads to more of the disease, the case for causality is strengthened. This would imply that those who had more severe cases of measles should be more likely to develop MS or to develop more serious symptoms earlier on. The evidence in this regard, however, is lacking. The biological gradient is seen most clearly with regard to environmental exposures. Newhouse, for instance, cited data gathered by Merewether and Prince that showed the relationship between length of employment in the asbestos industry and the incidence of fibrosis. The data look something like Figure 5-3. There seems to be a definite trend, in that longer exposure to asbestos results in a greater proportion of people who develop fibrosis.

For less obvious causal relationships there may be an amount of a toxic agent below which there are no adverse effects (at least none that we can measure with our current technology) and a ceiling, whereby no further increase leads to a greater effect. Some people postulate this is the case with ionizing radiation; there is no increased risk for cancer if exposure is below a certain threshold, whereas death is a certainty above an upper limit. Between these upper and lower limits, however, there may be a dose-response relationship.

Closely related to the idea of a dose-response relationship is that of an age-response relationship. Most disorders show a monotonic increase with age (e.g., Alzheimer's disease) or a decrease (measles), while a few may have a curvilinear relationship (the incidence of depression peaks in the 40s). In all cases, though, the age distribution should follow a plausible model, based on our knowledge of the disease process or previous findings. Any deviation should alert you that something else is going on. This was the case with Hodgkin's lymphoma, which showed an unusual pattern of peaking in the age range of 15–45, and then again in the mid-50s. Later research showed that there were actually two different subtypes.

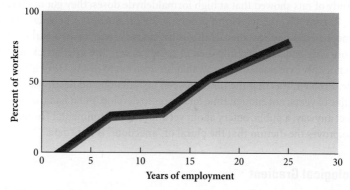

Figure 5-3. Length of employment in asbestos industry versus percent of workers who develop fibrosis. (From Newhouse M: Asbestos-related diseases: IV. Epidemiology of asbestos-related disease. In Michaels L, Chissick SS, editors: Asbestos: properties, applications, and hazards, vol 1, New York, 1979, Wiley.)

Biological Plausibility

If the association makes sense from the perspective of biology, there is a (somewhat) greater plausibility, if not probability, of a causal relationship. Thus, although the etiology of MS is still unknown, there is evidence from related disorders that viral infections, especially measles, can result in demyelination in the central nervous system. For example, high measles antibody titers are found in the serum and cerebrospinal fluid of patients with subacute sclerosing panencephalitis. This finding would indicate that a causal relationship between measles and MS is at least within the bounds of possibility.

However, a lack of plausibility may simply reflect our incomplete knowledge of physiology and biology. This may explain why people didn't bother to look for measles virus antigens in the gut; nobody expected them to be there. Until recently, no known mechanism existed to explain how psychologic stress could result in a greater susceptibility to infectious diseases and cancer. Only within the past few years has it been shown that stress may produce immune suppression by affecting immune cell function. As was the case with the criterion of specificity, plausibility strengthens the hypothesis, but a lack of plausibility does not weaken it.

Coherence

When discussing biologic plausibility, we noted that the absence of a plausible explanation was not necessarily damning to a good theory; it may simply reflect our ignorance. By the same token, the postulated causal relationship should not conflict with what *is* generally known about the disease or disorder.

For example, we mentioned that the prevalence of MS seemed to be proportional to the latitude, with some exceptions in Asia. However, the geographic distribution of measles is, if anything, opposite to what one would want; it is more common in the tropics than in more temperate climates. Using the criterion of coherence, this would argue against a causal link between the two diseases.

Needless to say, theories have been proposed to explain this inverse relationship. It has been postulated that subacute cases are common below the age of 15 years in the tropics and that this early infection provides protection against later, more serious ones. This may be taken as an example of Edington's Theory: "The number of different hypotheses erected to explain a given biologic phenomenon is inversely proportional to the available knowledge."

Experimental Evidence

In some cases there may be experimental evidence that can show a causal relationship. This evidence can be of many types: "true" experiments in the laboratory, randomized trials, animal models, experiments in nature, or interventions in which some preventative action is taken.

An experiment in nature would exist if a place were found where MS had been nonexistent until the society was introduced to the many benefits of civilization, including measles. This may indeed have been the case in the Faroe Islands. MS suddenly appeared in 1943, with 24 of 25 of the known cases first appearing between then and 1960, which is consistent with a mean age of onset of approximately 25 years. This "epidemic" coincided with the invasion of Denmark by Germany in 1940 and the subsequent stationing of approximately 800 British troops on the islands 4 days later. Although not conclusive evidence in its own right, this naturalistic experiment strengthens the case for MS being caused by some form of infectious agent.

Since an effective vaccine for measles was introduced to North America in 1963, there has been a dramatic decline in the prevalence of subacute sclerosing panencephalitis. If there is a causal relationship between measles and MS, we should have begun to see a similar drop in MS starting approximately 25 to 30 years later, or some time around 1990. (Unfortunately, just at the time we would have seen a decline, new brain imaging techniques, such as magnetic resonance imaging, were introduced, resulting in a sharp increase in detectable cases.) This would be an example of experimental evidence from an intervention. In this case, as in many others, the treatment was not predicated on an assumed relationship between the cause and effect; the aim of vaccination was simply to eliminate measles, not MS. Any evidence of a reduction in the incidence of MS would be a side benefit, probably unanticipated at the time the vaccination program began.

Experimental evidence again strengthens (but does not necessarily prove) causation. However, as with most of these criteria, its absence does not weaken the case because it is often extremely difficult or unethical to do the types of study that would yield less equivocal results.

Analogy

The weakest form of evidence regarding causality is arguing from an analogy. Returning again to the example of measles and subacute sclerosing panencephalitis, we can state that just as measles can cause one form of demyelinating disorder, it is reasonable to expect that it can cause another.

In this regard analogy is similar to biologic plausibility. For this reason, some authors don't distinguish between the two and drop this last category from the list of criteria for causality.

SUMMARY

Even if a theory passes all these criteria with flying colors, it does not necessarily *prove* causation beyond any shadow of a doubt. However, the more criteria that are met (especially the ones near the top of the list), the more likely it is that the causal hypothesis is in the right ball park, given the current state of our knowledge. Newer discoveries, however, may cause us to modify or even discard our cause-effect theory and to replace it with a different one. Buck notes that we would prefer a new hypothesis to a well-established one only if it meets at least one of the following criteria:

1. The new hypothesis makes more precise predictions than the old one.
2. More observations are explained with the new hypothesis.
3. Previous observations are explained in more detail.
4. The new hypothesis has passed tests that the older hypothesis has failed.
5. It suggests tests or makes predictions not made by the older hypothesis.
6. It has unified or connected phenomena not previously considered to be related.

Thus any causal hypothesis should be seen as just that: a hypothesis that accounts for what we know now but that may be modified or overturned at any time.

C.R.A.P. DETECTORS

C.R.A.P. Detectors V-1

Question. Ney used the statistic that the "rate of increase in child abuse parallels the rate of increase in abortions" to argue against abortions. Although he didn't calculate it, the correlation between the number of abortions and the number of cases of alleged physical ill treatment in Ontario between 1971 and 1977 is 0.85. Does this high correlation support Ney's case for a causal association?

Answer. One of the cardinal rules of statistics is that you can't draw causation from a correlation. In fact, we calculated that the correlation between the number of child abuse cases and the number of high school graduates during the same period is 0.86 and between cases of abuse and the gross revenue of Canadian railroads is 0.92. Nobody would argue, however, that the way to curb child abuse is to cut enrollment in high schools or to make the railroads lose money.

A nice demonstration that strong correlation does not necessarily imply any meaningful relationship is shown in Figure 5-4, which plots the number of wins in 1984 by teams in the American Football Conference as a function of the number of letters in the team name. The correlation between these two variables is 0.70, a figure high enough to cause most researchers to have dreams of tenure.

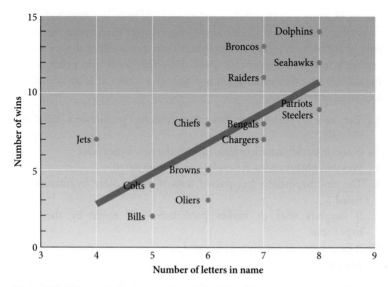

Figure 5-4. Relationship between number of wins by football teams and number of letters in their names.

C.R.A.P. Detectors V-2

Question. There has been concern expressed recently that the low rate of infection from measles has caused parents to become complacent and not have their children immunized. The fear is that there will be an outbreak of measles with the attending death rate that used to characterize the infection. Is this a concern? Was the vaccine responsible for the marked reduction in the case fatality rate from measles?

Answer. No, according to McKeown. Figure 5-5, based on the graph in his book *The Modern Rise of Population,* shows that the decline in the mortality rate from measles among children began long before the immunization program was initiated. This reflects the importance of establishing a temporal relationship before anything can be said about a causal one.

C.R.A.P. Detectors V-3

Question. A group of researchers in England found that bus drivers had a higher rate of coronary heart disease than did conductors. One hypothesis put forward to explain this was that conductors had to run up and down the stairs of the double-decker buses, whereas the drivers spent all day on their (and the buses') seats. Thus it may be that a more sedentary job increases the risk of heart disease. Is this a viable explanation for their results?

Answer. Only if all other differences between drivers and conductors are ruled out. The same research group compared the body builds of the two groups by doing an "epidemiologic survey" of their uniforms! As Figure 5-6 shows, a larger proportion of drivers than conductors had trouser waists of 36 inches or more, irrespective of age. So it would appear that there may have been constitutional differences between the groups from the very beginning, which makes an interpretation based on other group differences chancy at best.

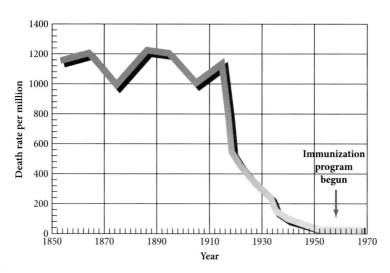

Figure 5-5. Mortality rate from measles through time. (Data from McKeown T: The modern rise of population, London, 1976, Edward Arnold.)

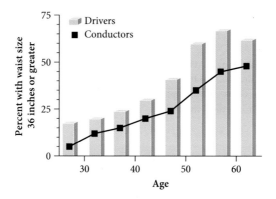

Figure 5-6. Waist sizes of conductors and drivers versus age.

REFERENCES

Elwood JM: *Causal relationships in medicine: a practical system for critical appraisal*, Oxford, 1987, Oxford University Press.

Fletcher RH, Fletcher SW, Wagner EH: *Clinical epidemiology: the essentials*, Baltimore, 1982, Williams & Wilkins.

Hill AB: The environment and disease: association or causation? *Proc R Soc Med* 58:295–300, 1965.

Whitaker JN: What causes the disease? In Scheinberg LC, editor: *Multiple sclerosis*, New York, 1983, Raven Press.

The Criteria

Strength of Association

Adams JM, Imagawa D: Measles antibodies in multiple sclerosis, *Proc Soc Exp Biol Med* 111:562–566, 1962.

Consistency of Association

Gray LA, Christopherson WM, Hoover RN: Estrogens and endometrial carcinoma, *Obstet Gynecol* 49:385–389, 1977.

Horwitz RI, Feinstein AR: Alternative analytic methods for case-control studies of estrogens and endometrial cancer, *N Engl J Med* 299:1089–1094, 1978.

Mack TM, Pike MC, Henderson BE: Estrogens and endometrial cancer in a retirement community, *N Engl J Med* 294:1262–1267, 1976.

McDonald TW, Annegers JF, O'Fallon WM: Exogenous estrogen and endometrial carcinoma: case-control and incidence study, *Am J Obstet Gynecol* 127:572–580, 1977.

Norrby E: Viral antibodies in multiple sclerosis, *Prog Med Virol* 24:1–39, 1978.

Smith DC, Prentice R, Thompson DJ: Association of exogenous estrogens and endometrial carcinoma, *N Engl J Med* 293:1164–1167, 1975.

Ziel HK, Finkle WD: Increased risk of endometrial carcinoma among users of conjugated estrogens, *N Engl J Med* 293:1167–1170, 1975.

Specificity of Association

Buchanan WD: Asbestos-related diseases: I. Introduction. In Michaels L, Chissick SS, editors: *Asbestos: properties, applications, and hazards*, vol 1, New York, 1979, Wiley.

McDonald JC, McDonald AD: Epidemiology of mesothelioma from estimated incidence, *Prev Med* 6:426–446, 1977.

Pertschuk LP, Cook AW, Gupta J: Measles antigen in multiple sclerosis: identification in the jejunum by immunofluorescence, *Life Sci* 19:1603–1608, 1976.

Temporality of Association

Barker DJ, Eriksson JG, Osmond C: Fetal origins of adult disease: strength of effects and biological basis, *Int J Epidemiol* 31:1235–1239, 2002.

Dyer AR: A method for combining results from several prospective epidemiological studies, *Stat Med* 5:303–317, 1986.

Eisenberg L: The fathers of autistic children, *Am J Orthopsychiatry* 27:715–724, 1957.

Eisenberg L, Kanner L: Early infantile autism 1943–55, *Am J Orthopsychiatry* 26:556–566, 1956.

Pitfield M, Oppenheim AN: Child rearing attitudes of mothers of psychotic children, *J Child Psychol Psychiatry* 5:51–57, 1964.

Biological Gradient

Newhouse M: Asbestos-related diseases: IV. Epidemiology of asbestos-related disease. In Michaels L, Chissick SS, editors: *Asbestos: properties, applications, and hazards,* vol 1, New York, 1979, Wiley.

Biological Plausibility

Marx JL: The immune system "belongs in the body" *Science* 227:1190–1192, 1985.

ter Meulen V, Stephenson JR: The possible role of viral infections in multiple sclerosis and other related demyelinating diseases. In Hallpike JF, Adams CWM, Tourtelloutte WW, editors: *Multiple sclerosis: pathology, diagnosis and management,* London, 1983, Chapman & Hall.

Coherence

Bloch A: *Murphy's law, and other reasons why things go wrong,* Los Angeles, 1979, Prince/Stern/Sloan.

Carp RI, Warner HB, Merz GS: Viral etiology of multiple sclerosis, *Prog Med Virol* 24:158–177, 1978.

Experimental Evidence

Bloch AB, Orenstein WA, Wassilak SG: Epidemiology of measles and its complications. In Gruenberg EM, Lewis C, Goldston SE, editors: *Vaccinating against brain syndromes: the campaign against measles and rubella,* New York, 1986, Oxford University Press.

Kurtzke JF, Hyllested K: Multiple sclerosis in the Faroe Islands: I. Clinical and epidemiological features, *Ann Neurol* 5:6–21, 1979.

Summary

Buck C: Popper's philosophy for epidemiologists, *Int J Epidemiol* 4:159–168, 1975.

C.R.A.P. Detectors

McKeown T: *The modern rise of population,* London, 1976, Edward Arnold.

Morris JN, Heady JA, Raffle PAB. Physique of London busmen: epidemiology of uniforms. *Lancet,* Sept. 15, 1956:569–570.

Morris JN, Heady JA, Raffle PAB et al: Coronary heart-disease and physical activity of work, *Lancet.* Nov 21, 1953:1053–1057.

Ney P: Relationship between abortion and child abuse, *Can J Psychiatry* 24:10–12, 1979.

TO READ FURTHER

Department of Clinical Epidemiology and Biostatistics: How to read clinical journals: IV. To determine etiology or causation, *Can Med Assoc J* 124:985–990,1981.

Hill AB: The environment and disease: association or causation? *Proc R Soc Med* 58:295–300, 1965.

6

Ethics

Before 1945, it was not at all unusual for patients to be enrolled in experiments without their consent and sometimes even without their knowledge of being subjects in a study. Medicine was much more paternalistic then, and it was assumed that physicians would look after the best interests of their patients. That view of the world was one of the casualties of World War II when it was discovered that physicians, with real medical degrees, performed horrific "experiments" on concentration camp inmates in Europe. Later, gross violations of patients' rights came to light in the United States and other countries, some involving studies done in the past, but more disturbingly, a few of recent vintage. Some of the most notable historical examples include experiments (1) at the Tuskegee Institute, where 400 poor, uneducated black men were given heavy metals or placebo for their syphilis even after penicillin was discovered; (2) at the Willowbrook State school, where retarded children were admitted only if their parents enrolled them in a U.S. Army study of gamma globulin after they were deliberately infected with hepatitis; and (3) at the Sloan-Kettering Cancer Research Institute, where live cancer cells were injected into old, chronically ill patients without their knowledge. More recent examples include an experiment at the University of California at Los Angeles that involved taking schizophrenic patients off their maintenance medication, which resulted in the suicide of at least one person, and the Central Intelligence Agency–sponsored research at the Montreal Neurological Institute on the effectiveness of lysergic acid diethylamide (LSD) and sensory deprivation on "brainwashing."

The first formal attempt at trying to prevent the misuse of research subjects was the **Nuremberg Code**, drafted immediately after World War II. Through the years, this standard was modified a number of times, as in the World Health Organization's **Declarations of Helsinki**, and now all major granting agencies and professional organizations in the developed countries have their own codes. Despite differences in wording and emphasis, the central concept in all of these standards is the same: the *autonomy of the individual.* This seemingly innocuous phase, which means that each person should be the master of his of her fate, has many implications.

173

The first is that the person has to *consent* to take part in the study. Consent is meaningless, though, unless the person understands what it is he or she is consenting to; thus there has to be *informed consent*. Finally, informed consent isn't of much use if the person does not have the ability to refuse, so the phrase that is now commonly used is *free and informed consent*. Let's take a closer look at what these terms imply.

FREELY GIVEN CONSENT

It appears obvious that coercing people into serving as research subjects is patently unethical and nothing that we as researchers would ever do. But consider the following situations:

1. You are the local investigator in a multicenter trial to determine the usefulness of antibiotics in treating ulcers. You ask the next 30 patients attending your outpatient clinic who meet the criteria to participate in this study, assuring them that their future care will not be jeopardized if they refuse. To reimburse you for your time in filling out the required forms, you will be paid $500 for each person who completes the trial.
2. To study the effects of immobility on muscle fibers, you want to have otherwise healthy volunteers wear a cast on their nondominant arm for 6 weeks. You advertise in the college newspaper and offer to pay subjects $150 a week.
3. You want to compare the efficacy of heat therapy versus acupuncture in patients with rotator cuff injury. To improve compliance during the 10-week trial, you will remunerate subjects after they have completed all 20 sessions.
4. It is hypothesized that allergic reactions can be classically conditioned by exposing subjects to an allergen in the presence of a previously neutral stimulus. You try this with 20 students enrolled in an introductory psychology class who must participate in 3 hours of studies to meet the course requirements.

Coercion

Each of these studies, which are based on actual proposals, raises concerns about the subjects' freedom to say "No." Although reassured that refusal will not jeopardize their future care, patients may still have concerns that not participating in a study will anger their physician, resulting in second-rate care. This puts subtle pressure on them to sign up, despite any misgivings they may have about being in the study. Further, there is a power imbalance between the physician and the patient that raises at least the potential for abuse and a violation of the therapeutic alliance. To avoid this, whenever possible, clinicians should not enlist their own patients in studies but should delegate the task to another person (e.g., colleague, resident, nurse). On occasion, this may present a dilemma because the attending physician may be the person who could best explain the study to the potential subject and address any questions or concerns. In these circumstances, it would be best if the clinician informs the patient about the details of the study but leaves the room when consent is sought by the other person overseeing the experiment.

Although the use of indentured servants was officially abolished in the United States well over 100 years ago, pockets of it still exist in the form of psychology students, postdoctoral fellows, and laboratory technicians who supply a disproportionate amount of information about "human" behavior and blood for new assays. The reasons for this are obvious: these people are generally compliant and available, often in large numbers. However, the problems with using them are similar to those outlined in the previous paragraph. If participation in a certain number of studies is a course requirement, then refusing can lead to a lower grade. Technicians and fellows don't want to jeopardize their current jobs or their chances of future ones by alienating their boss, who also may be the writer of a needed letter of reference. The American Psychological Association stipulates that students should be offered an alternative to participating in research studies, such as writing a paper. Laboratory supervisors should act like attending physicians and never ask people who are beholden to them to take part in an experiment or even to donate blood. To do otherwise would strain the freedom of refusal.

Payment to Physicians

Paying a physician more than a token amount to enroll patients in a study and complete the required forms is problematic at the best of times. In some studies, these "bounty fees" can be as much as a few thousand dollars a patient, which far exceeds the remuneration for the time spent doing these tasks and raises the question of whose interests the physician is serving. If there is the slightest possibility that tests or other procedures will be performed to determine eligibility for a study and not because the patient requires them, or that diagnoses may be subtly modified to meet study criteria (as happened in a recent breast cancer trial), then ethical practice is jeopardized. Even worse is making the fee contingent on the patient completing the trial, which puts the doctor in a situation of even greater conflict of interest. There should not be any financial disincentive to removing a patient from a trial because of adverse reactions; even the perception that this may occur should be avoided. Furthermore, the *National Council on Bioethics in Human Research* states explicitly that "patients should know of financial arrangements concerning trials." Whether the researcher will receive money, or a personal computer, or a fax machine are deemed "material facts that a research participant would need to know."

Payment to Subjects

In a similar fashion, paying the subjects only after they complete a long series of procedures may put undue pressure on them to continue in the study after the point at which they would otherwise say "Enouugh, already." From both a scientific and a logistic point of view, we would like all subjects who are enrolled to stay in the study until the end; otherwise, we as researchers are plagued with missing data, fewer subjects than we need, and threats to the validity of the study. However, these very real methodologic considerations should not override the subject's freedom to withdraw at any time. One compromise is to pay patients on a sliding schedule, which is a larger amount the longer they stay in the study.

This raises the related issue of how much to pay subjects in the first place. We don't work for free (although we may feel grossly underpaid and undervalued), so why should we expect strangers to volunteer their time for the benefit of our research? The delicate balancing act is to find an amount that would reimburse subjects for their time, effort, and discomfort but not so much that they would take risks or jeopardize their health simply for the money. In the real world, we *do* pay people more do risky jobs that we wouldn't do ourselves—build or paint bridges, repair industrial chimneys, or fight forest fires. In the world of research however, we should not coerce people into participating in studies in which we ourselves would not enroll. In most places we're familiar with, if subjects are paid at all, the going rate is slightly above the minimum wage (plus traveling and parking expenses, if required), but this can be increased slightly if some discomfort is involved, such as venipuncture or swallowing a nasogastric tube. However, in many clinical trials, patients are not paid for participating.

INFORMED CONSENT

Elements of Consent

Before people can agree to participate in a study, they must know what the study is about and what it is that they're agreeing to so the process of informing the potential subject is central to ethical consent. All too often, researchers regard the written *consent form* as if it were the same as *informed consent,* but as we'll see, the two are not always the same. Before you would volunteer to be in a study, what would you want to know? Most likely, it would include the following:

1. The researchers and the sponsoring institutions or companies.
2. The title of the project.

3. The overall purpose of the study.

4. A description of what's going to happen to you (e.g., having blood drawn or a device inserted into one unmentionable orifice or another, being interviewed about your habits, etc.); what you will be expected to do or not do (e.g., filling out forms, taking medications, avoiding products with aspirin, lifting weights etc.); how often these things will happen; and how long each session and the whole study will last. If the treatment you receive (or may not receive in a placebo-controlled study) will be determined randomly, you would definitely want to know this.

5. The risks and the probabilities of the risks occurring. You likely don't want to hear about relatively innocuous or minor problems, especially if they don't happen often. What you do want to know are which ones occur relatively often (which means at least 5% of the time) and those that may be rarer but are potentially more severe. These two factors—frequency and severity—act in a reciprocal way: adverse reactions should be mentioned (with their probabilities) if they are rare but severe or less severe but more frequent.

6. Any possible benefit from participating in the study, such as having a thorough work-up, getting a potentially useful treatment or having access to a drug that would not otherwise be available. However, this must be counterbalanced by the fact that there is a chance you may get a placebo, or that the new therapy may not work as well as the standard, or even that the experimental treatment may do some harm.

7. You would want some assurance that your test results will be confidential; for instance, if any publication comes out of this, you will not be identifiable by name or on the basis of personal characteristics, and no one outside the team would have access to your records. This may have to be abrogated under some circumstances. For example, most drug companies reserve the right for them or the national drug safety agency to review individual records with the person's name attached to minimize the possibility of fraud by the researchers. If this is the case, you'd want to know.

8. If you were a patient, you would want assurance that you could refuse to participate or agree and change your mind later, even in the middle of the study, without affecting any care you may require in the future. You may not believe this assurance, but it would be nice to get it in any case.

9. Whom you can contact if you have any questions about the study or if an emergency develops.

10. Most importantly, how much you're going to get paid for doing all this or if you're not going to be paid at all.

These are the basic elements of informed consent. Often a form that contains all these features is signed and kept by the researcher, but this is as much for legal purposes as ethical. From an ethical perspective, what is important is the information, not the form. It could be the case that the best way to convey this information may be with a separate information sheet or a videotape, or orally, or in a "comic-book" format with the form simply stating, "I saw the tape, understood it, and here's my signature." The advantage of a written consent form or information sheet, especially for trials of a new therapy, is that the person can take it home and discuss it with his or her physician or family members before agreeing to be a participant.

Language of Consent

Being in the health care business immediately implies two things: (1) we have at least a university education, and (2) we have our own jargon, tossing around terms like "lesion," "pruritus," or "range of motion" as if we know what it is we're talking about. The average person, though, uses a language rarely spoken by us professional types—something called English. In this strange language, the red stuff in our veins is "blood," not "serum"; the organ that pumps it around is the "heart," not the "myocardium"; and "shock" is what happens when you touch a live wire or hear that your worst enemy won the lottery. Moreover, it's been estimated that the typical person on the street who has a high school education actually reads at approximately the level of a sixth grader. What this means is that you or your colleague should not be the ones to decide whether the form is understandable to the lay public; neither should it be your secretary, for that matter, because he or she most likely has been exposed to this jargon as long as you have (and can probably spell the words better). Any information conveyed to the potential subjects should be reviewed by a group of people with comparable backgrounds and checked for comprehension and readability. Additionally, a number of computerized spell-checking programs can estimate the reading level necessary to understand the material; if it's above the sixth grade, rewrite the form.

Special Groups

Getting informed consent is especially problematic with three groups of people: (1) children; (2) those whose cognitive abilities may be compromised because of retardation, dementia, or psychosis; and (3) those from a cultural background different from the majority of people. Some people have argued that these people should not be used in studies at all because they cannot give meaningful consent. However, adopting this viewpoint would result in "therapeutic orphans"—groups for which potentially useful diagnostic tests or treatments cannot be developed because the individuals would be excluded from investigation. Rather, it would make more sense to develop strategies that would minimize any potential problem.

The usual procedure used with children is to get consent from their parents. If the child is old enough to understand what is happening (an undefined age, which depends more on mental maturity than age), then his or her assent (i.e., acceptance not necessarily accompanied by a signed form) must also be obtained, and the child's "No" always overrides the parents' "Yes." But there are limits to what parents can consent to in the name of their children, which vary from one set of ethical standards to another. One of the clearest statements is from the Medical Research Council of Canada, which states the following:

> A relevant measure is that society and parents should not expose children to greater risks, for the sake of pure medical research [i.e., the child does not stand to gain from any therapeutic intervention], than the children take in their everyday lives. Parents control this level of exposure now. . . . They may permit others to handle their children in ways that would otherwise constitute a technical and minor legal assault, but not where pain or discomfort beyond carefully defined limits would be liable to occur.

The problems in gaining consent from incompetent adult patients are in many ways similar to those with children; it cannot always be assumed that the people understand what is being asked of them and that their signature implies informed consent. By the same token, some of these people may be capable of comprehending at least part of the information, and most would have been mentally and legally competent adults at some point in their lives. Thus decisions must be made on a case-by-case basis, rather than seeing them as a homogeneous group. If there is an official guardian or a close family member, it is assumed that this person knows what the patient would have wanted if he or she were competent and will keep the patient's best interests uppermost when deciding for the person. However, if the patient has been in an institution for any length of time, it is possible that the family may not be involved any more or may no longer be sensitive to the personality and preferences of the patient. In the past, hospital administrators played the part of the family member when none was available, but this is becoming less and less acceptable each year. Because they may have a vested interest in seeing research conducted within the institution (especially if they are allowed to charge the granting agency for "overhead"), administrators are in a conflict-of-interest situation. Some jurisdictions are moving toward government-appointed surrogate decision makers, but these laws are still new and highly variable from one place to another.

Research involving people from different cultural backgrounds raises a number of difficulties. The most obvious, and perhaps the easiest to deal with, is that their primary language may not be English. The information about the study must be translated, using the usual techniques to ensure the adequacy of the translation, ideally by someone who is familiar with culturally appropriate ways of expressing the terms and concepts. (Be aware of the fact that "culture" means more than a shared language. In Mexican Spanish, for example, *comadre* can be used on a consent form to refer to a close personal friend or an advisor. In Nicaragua, though, the closeness is too close; a *comadre* is "the other woman.") A more difficult problem is that standards of ethical practice are not universal but vary widely from one cultural group to another even within the same country. For example, the usual way of introducing a randomized controlled trial (RCT) to potential subjects is for the clinician to say something along the lines of "We don't know if treatment A is any better than treatment B, so the one you get will be decided by the flip of a coin." However, it is inconceivable in many Far Eastern cultures for physicians to say "I don't know"—they would never say it, and patients would never want to hear it. Consequently, for a study involving these groups to succeed, it may be necessary to have one consent form for the majority culture and another for people from other backgrounds, even within the same city.

The delicate balancing act is respecting the viewpoints of people from different backgrounds while not doing violence to our own code of ethics. In some cultural groups, for instance, it would be unthinkable for an individual to agree or decline participation in a trial without the express approval of the community leader. But even though the leader's consent is sufficient within that group, our standards require individual consent, meaning that we would have to obtain both the leader's permission to comply with the group's mores and the individual's agreement to comply with our own ethical code.

When Consent Need Not Be Written

There are a few situations where the consent may be obtained verbally, and a written form is not needed. The most common situation is when the person is asked to complete a questionnaire. As long as it is clearly indicated to the subjects that it is part of research study and that they can omit any items that they may find offensive, then written consent is superfluous. If the person does not want to be a part of the study, then he or she can simply throw the questionnaire away, leave out objectionable items, or return the whole thing entirely blank. In other words, completing the form is implicit consent.

Other examples, which may vary from one institution to another, are drawn from a list complied by the Office for Protection from Research

Risks of the National Institutes of Health that outlines research activities that may have "expedited review procedures"; that is, procedures can be reviewed only by the chair or "one of the more experienced reviewers" of the Institutional Review Board (IRB). These are procedures that involve "no more than minimal risk" and include (1) noninvasive recording procedures involving at most insignificant amounts of energy (e.g., electrocardiograms, electroencephalogram tests of sensory acuity, weighing, or detection of naturally occurring radioactivity, but not the use of x-rays or microwaves), (2) moderate exercise by healthy volunteers, or (3) studies of perception or cognition where the subject's behavior is not manipulated and there is no stress.

When Consent Need Not Be Obtained

Consent forms can be formidable and look almost like legal documents with room for signatures, dates, witnesses, and the like. Sometimes the anxiety produced by asking someone to read and sign it may be greater than any possible harm from being in the study. Harmless research would include studies that use "pathologic waste," such as the placenta, tissue removed during an operation, excreta, or another 5 to 10 ml of blood after the needle was inserted for clinical purposes. Here, consent may be waived entirely by the IRB. Some thorny issues have arisen regarding who benefits financially if the research done on such material leads to profitable diagnostic tests or cell lines, but we'll leave that to the lawyers.

Other research that does not require consent or IRB review are (1) studies that compare one educational intervention against another and those that involve the use of educational tests (presumably under the assumption that students are fair game for anything or that nothing works in education, in any case); (2) surveys or observational studies where the individual cannot be identified on any of the forms; or (3) studies that use medical records, again with the proviso that the data are recorded in such a way that an outsider would be unable to identify who the patient is.

A last area where consent is not needed (or at least, not obtained) is more invasive than the previous examples and involves situations where it is impossible to gain consent. For example, studies comparing different resuscitation strategies for sudden death obviously cannot enroll patients ahead of time, and it is, by definition, problematic to get signed consent from someone who has just died. A bit more troublesome are situations where consent can be gained, but the time delay may preclude this. For example, some interventions with extremely low birth weight children or other neonates at high risk have to be started within minutes of birth. By the time the study is explained to the parents and a consent form is signed, it is too late for the experimental treatment to work. The options are either (1) gaining consent from all potential parents ahead of time, (2) not doing the study, or (3) doing it without prior consent. The first option means that potentially useful treatments will not be introduced; and the third option, the one we favor, raises the old issue of medical paternalism.

OTHER ISSUES

Ethics and Methodology

Some IRBs see themselves as research ethics committees, stating that they are concerned solely with the ethical components of the study (e.g., informed consent, confidentiality) and not with the methodologic aspects. Most committees, though, see methodologic rigor and ethics as inextricably interwoven. The reasoning behind the belief that a badly designed ethical study is an oxymoron is that if the research is flawed in a significant way, then its chances of producing usable, meaningful information are close to zero, so there cannot be any potential gain to the subject or to society to balance against any possible risk. The corollary to this is that the more invasive the procedures used, the more rigorous the study has to be. We could tolerate a relatively weak design when all the subjects have to do is fill out a questionnaire, but a far tighter design must be used if the study involves inserting a catheter into the person.

This does not give license to researchers to do truly Mickey Mouse studies if they are relatively benign; there is still the ethical issue of producing data that are unreliable but that may be accepted as facts by people not aware of the limitations of the methodology. The prime example is the "reports" of the sexual behavior of people that appear in magazines and even books. Questionnaires are often distributed through truly haphazard means, response rates rarely exceed 2%, and no checks are made for people with strong views sending in two, three, or a dozen forms. On the basis of these travesties, myths about the frequency of intercourse, the number of people having affairs, and the like become accepted as facts. Here's the bottom line: bad research is unethical.

Role of Uncertainty

All research is based on ignorance. If we know ahead of time what the outcome will be, we shouldn't be doing the study. (As you can see, "ignorance" extends only as far as the results; it should not include the methods or analysis.) Let's take a look at both sides of this issue.

Some clinicians won't enroll their patients in a study because they "know," or at least strongly suspect, that treatment A is better than B or that this specific patient would benefit more from one treatment than another. In the absence of objective data supporting these beliefs, this is one area where a bit of ignorance (or at least humility) may be worthwhile. It's not necessary to recount here all the instances of therapies that were believed to be effective and later turned out to be totally useless or even harmful.

The converse, though, is that if the researcher has a well-founded belief that one treatment *is* better than another, it would be patently unethical to do a study in which some of the patients get a less effective intervention. In any trial of two or more methods (diagnostic, therapeutic, or the like, and where one procedure may in fact be a placebo), the patients in the study must only be those *for whom there is uncertainty* about which arm of the trial would be the most appropriate. Sometimes, it is known beforehand that one treatment is more effective than another or one diagnostic test more sensitive than the alternative. A trial would be justified in these circumstances if the less effective alternative also had fewer adverse effects. From an ethical point of view, the question (as always) is whether the benefit to the patient outweighs the possible harm.

Ethics of Placebo Controls

If it is known that one treatment is effective for a certain condition, is it ever ethical to test a different treatment for that condition against a placebo, or does this violate the principle of uncertainty we've just been discussing? Some prominent researchers have argued that denying patients an effective treatment violates the Declaration of Helsinki, which states that "every patient—including those of a control group, if any—should be assured of the best proven diagostic and therapeutic method." Even the person who popularized the modern clinical trial, Bradford Hill, said that if a treatment already exists "the doctor will wish to know whether a new treatment is more, or less, effective than the old, not that it is more effective than nothing."

Well, not all doctors. The Food and Drug Administration (FDA) in the United States, for instance, requires that any new nonsteroidal anti-inflammatory drug (NSAID) be tested against a placebo, even though many NSAIDs exist (approximately one for every three arthritis patients, it seems). Is the FDA just being bureaucratic, or are there valid reasons for having a placebo group, even when there is an effective therapy? The answer is "Yes."

In fact, most textbooks see a placebo group as de rigueur even when a proven therapy exists. To explain the reasons, let's imagine a two-arm trial of a new drug, Moreprophet, versus the well-established acetylsalicylic acid (ASA) for the treatment of rheumatoid arthritis. What are the possible outcomes? First, Moreprophet could be significantly better than ASA, resulting in much more profit for the drug company. Secondly, it could be significantly worse, leading the executives of the company to down large

amounts of ASA for their headaches. What is more likely, in these days of
lookalike drugs, is that there is no appreciable difference. Now what are the
possible reasons for the lack of difference? The first is that the drugs really
are not all that different in anything except price, and we would be correct
in staying with the cheaper ASA. The next reason is that one drug actually is
better than the other, but the trial wasn't large enough to detect a difference;
in essence, a Type II error. Last, the drugs may be different and there may
have been enough subjects, but the study was badly designed or executed—
poorly chosen and insensitive outcome measures, badly trained raters, non-
compliant patients, or a host of other factors. In this case, because there is
no placebo arm with which to compare the results, it is impossible to know
if both drugs were equally effective or were equally ineffective *in the hands
of this research team*. If the ASA group did not do any better than a placebo
group, though, it would have signaled to us that the study was flawed, and
we shouldn't trust the results.

Another reason for a placebo group was seen in a recent trial of flosequinan for treating heart failure. When it was compared with an angio-
tensin converting enzyme (ACE) inhibitor, the two were found to be equally
efficacious, which would indicate that it is an acceptable substitute, especially if it were cheaper. When either flosequinan or placebo were given to
patients receiving an established therapy, though, a different story emerged;
it significantly increased the risk of death.

A third reason in favor of comparing a new treatment against a placebo
rather than an alternative is that, paradoxically, fewer people are put at risk
of adverse drug reactions (ADRs). Let's assume that ADRs occur 10% of the
time with both drugs. When we compare an active drug against a placebo,
then we usually expect a fairly large difference, so the sample size needs to
be relatively small; say, 50 patients per group. This means that nobody in
the placebo group will have an ADR, and five patients in the new treatment
group will. Now, if we compare the new treatment against an established
one, the difference between the two will be much smaller, so that a far larger
sample size is needed; say, 100 per group. In this case, 10 patients in each
group will experience ADRs, four times the number in a placebo-controlled
trial. Thus, it may actually be *more* ethical to use a placebo comparison
rather than an active control group.

A final objection to the placebo group is that it always deprives half
the patients of receiving an effective therapy. If the new drug is compared
with standard therapy and the new drug works, then all patients receive
some benefit; if it doesn't work, at least half have gotten something effective.
In a placebo trial, if the treatment works, half benefit; if it doesn't work,
nobody gets anything effective. With this logic, it would always be better to
omit the placebo arm. However, this assumes that all treatments are safe.
As we saw with flosequinan and many other drugs, side effects do exist and

can sometimes be fatal, even for accepted treatments. Those in the placebo group may not enjoy the benefits of treatment, but by the same token, they are not subjected to the risks.

So what's the bottom line? If the disease is life-threatening or may result in irreversible injury and a proven therapy exists, there is no issue; a placebo group would be patently unethical. At the opposite extreme, if the disease is relatively benign, and the placebo patients are simply delayed in receiving a proven therapy for a few days or weeks, there are likely few ethical concerns with using a placebo group. The problem, as always, lies in the middle. Here the balance is between the risk of allowing a disease to remain untreated for a given length of time, versus the benefit of measuring the exact effect of the treatment, as opposed to its effect relative to some other intervention and having more confidence in results showing equivalence. As the risk and the interval increase, the balance is tipped toward using only an active comparison; as the risk and duration of the trial decrease, the direction is toward a placebo arm. The result of this calculus is highly subjective and dependent on the local IRB.

REFERENCES

American Psychological Association: Ethical principles of psychologists and code of conduct, *Am Psychol* 47:1597–1611, 1992.

Cowley AJ, Wynne RD, Swami A: A comparison of the effects of captopril and flosequinan in patients with severe heart failure, *Cardiovasc Drugs Ther* 6:465–470, 1992.

Hill AB: Medical ethics and controlled trials, *Br Med J* 1:1043–1049, 1963.

Medical Research Council of Canada: *Guidelines on research involving human subjects,* Ottawa, 1987, MRC.

NCBHR Office: Divided loyalties: an anthology of conflict of interest duties, *NCBHR Communiqué* 6:11–16, 1995.

Office for Protection from Research Risks: *Exempt research and research that may undergo expedited review,* OPRR Reports, No. 95–02, Rockville MD, National Institutes of Health, 1995.

Office for Protection from Research Risks: *Protection of human subjects,* OPRR Reports, Code of Federal Regulation 45 CFR 46, Rockville MD, National Institutes of Health, 1983.

Packer M, Rouleau J, Swedberg K: Effect of flosequinan on survival in chronic heart failure: preliminary results of the PROFILE study, *Circulation* 88:(suppl I):301, 1993 (Abstract).

Rothman KJ, Michels KB: The continuing unethical use of placebo controls, *N Engl J Med* 331:394–398, 1994.

Streincr DL: The ethics of placebo-controlled trials, *Can J Psychiatry* 40:165–166, 1995 (editorial).

Streiner DL: The lesser of two evils: the ethics of placebo-controlled trials. *Can J Psychiatry* 53:430–432, 2008.

TO READ FURTHER

Beauchamp TL, Childress JF: *Principles of biomedical ethics,* ed 3, New York, 1989, Oxford University Press.

Klerman GL: Scientific and ethical considerations in the use of placebo controls in clinical trials in psychopharmacology, *Psychopharcacol Bull* 22:25–29, 1986.

Levine R: *Ethics and regulations of clinical research,* ed 2, Baltimore, 1986, Urban and Schwarzenber.

Appendix

A BRIEF EPIDEMISH-ENGLISH DICTIONARY

In the course of writing their reports and journal articles, researchers in epidemiology often use words or phrases whose meanings are somewhat obscure. To assist the reader in understanding these terms (and to provide a little amusement), we provide herein a brief dictionary.

To begin, we offer the definition of clinical epidemiology (itself an obscure term), which is credited to Dr. Stephen Leader of the University of Sydney:

> "Clinical epidemiology is that branch of alchemy whose goal it is to turn bulls—t into airline tickets."

And now to the dictionary.

When The Researcher Says	He or She Really Means
A trend was noted.	The statistical test was not significant.
The demographic characteristics of the nonresponders were similar to those of the rest of the sample.	All we really had on them were age and sex.
Agreement between the raters was acceptable.	The agreement was so bad that we don't dare to include the actual number in the paper.
The questionnaire was circulated to a panel of experts to establish face validity.	Our friends liked it . . . and the bottle of scotch we included.
The rate of lung cancer among the hourly rate employees was significantly higher, which may be caused by excess PCBP exposure.	It might also be caused by obvious things like smoking and social class, but I'm interested in PCBP today.

In a case series of 12 patients, 9 showed clinically significant improvement on the experimental drug.

With the help of the drug company representative, I judged which patients got better under my care.

The correlation was highly significant (p < 0.0001).

With 10,000 subjects, *any* correlation is highly significant.

The response rate was 60%, which is acceptable for studies of this type.

However, the study itself was so bad that even a 100% response rate wouldn't have saved it.

Although there was no overall difference in mortality, the rate of left clavicular cancer was higher in blue-eyed women in the exposed group.

If you look at enough things, sooner or later one of them is bound to turn out to be significantly different.

Although the results appear to be consistent with the predictions, further research is warranted.

I've already applied for a new grant this year.

Further research is required to clarify the results.

I haven't a clue what it all means.

The difference was statistically significant (p < 0.0001) . . .

. . . but clinically useless.

The study was a single-blind trial.

Everybody knew who was getting what except the poor patient.

A retrospective study was conducted.

We had all these data sitting around and needed some fast publications.

Morbidity and mortality from Streinorman's disease represents a significant burden on society.

It's my own narrow interest, but I have to justify the research somehow.

The overall agreement was 87%, which represents a truly remarkable rate of agreement ($\kappa = 0.12$).

Chance-corrected agreement was so abysmal that we thought we had better talk about raw agreement.

Based on current trends, the incidence of self-pollution in the year 2010 will be . . .

Draw a straight line through the data from one hospital in 1990 and 2000, and that's what we got.

It is widely known that . . .

I can't be bothered to look up the reference.

A one-tailed test was used.

The results wouldn't be significant with a two-tailed test.

After adjusting for baseline differences between the groups . . .

We did a lousy job of randomizing.

After adjusting for confounders . . .

Boy, did these groups differ!

One possible explanation for these results is . . .

I can only think of one.

Forty patients agreed to participate.

The others were able to pay their hospital bills.

After conducting a pilot study, we decided to use a mailed questionnaire.

We got tired of people slamming the phone in our ear.

After conducting a pilot study, we decided to use face-to-face interviews.

They wouldn't return the mailed questionnaires either.

The data were normalized by truncating outliers.

We couldn't get the results we wanted, so we threw out subjects until we got what we were looking for.

We did not include premorbid status and number of previous hospitalizations in the model.

We forgot to gather these data.

The agreement between raters was:
  excellent
  good
  acceptable
  low

The agreement between raters was:
  good
  fair
  nonexistent
  negative

Data were analyzed using the Schmedlap-Scheisskopf test.

We tried the usual tests, but they didn't give significant results.

A fiducial reference line . . .

A scratch

Although it has not been possible to provide definite answers to these questions . . .

The experiment didn't work out, but I figured I could at least get a publication out of it.

Three of the samples were chosen for detailed study.

None of the other samples worked, so we threw them out.

Correct within an order of magnitude

Wrong

The assays were handled with extreme care during the experiments.

We didn't drop any on the floor.

No one has looked at this before.

Nobody else really cares about this.

Time and time again . . .

I've seen two cases.

In case after case after case . . .

I've seen three cases.

Index